Post-Traumatic Stress Disorder

Disorder

A Clinician's Guide

The Plenum Series on Stress and Coping

Series Editor:

Donald Meichenbaum, *University of Waterloo, Waterloo, Ontario, Canada*

Editorial Board: Bruce P. Dohrenwend, *Columbia University*
Marianne Frankenhaeuser, *University of Stockholm*
Norman Garmezy, *University of Minnesota*
Mardi J. Horowitz, *University of California Medical School, San Francisco*
Richard S. Lazarus, *University of California, Berkeley*
Michael Rutter, *University of London*
Dennis C. Turk, *University of Pittsburgh*
John P. Wilson, *Cleveland State University*
Camille Wortman, *University of Michigan*

A CLINICAL GUIDE TO THE TREATMENT OF THE
HUMAN STRESS RESPONSE
George S. Everly, Jr.

COPING WITH LIFE CRISES
An Integrated Approach
Edited by Rudolf H. Moos

COPING WITH NEGATIVE LIFE EVENTS
Clinical and Social Psychological Perspectives
Edited by C. R. Snyder and Carol E. Ford

DYNAMICS OF STRESS
Physiological, Psychological, and Social Perspectives
Edited by Mortimer H. Appley and Richard Trumbull

HUMAN ADAPTATION TO EXTREME STRESS
From the Holocaust to Vietnam
Edited by John P. Wilson, Zev Harel, and Boaz Kahana

INTERNATIONAL HANDBOOK OF TRAUMATIC STRESS SYNDROMES
Edited by John P. Wilson and Beverley Raphael

POST-TRAUMATIC STRESS DISORDER
A Clinician's Guide
Kirtland C. Peterson, Maurice F. Prout, and Robert A. Schwarz

THE SOCIAL CONTEXT OF COPING
Edited by John Eckenrode

STRESS BETWEEN WORK AND FAMILY
Edited by John Eckenrode and Susan Gore

WOMEN, WORK, AND HEALTH
Edited by Marianne Frankenhaeuser, Ulf Lundberg, and Margaret Chesney

A Continuation Order Plan is available for this series. A continuation order will bring delivery of each new volume immediately upon publication. Volumes are billed only upon actual shipment. For further information please contact the publisher.

Post-Traumatic Stress Disorder

Disorder

A Clinician's Guide

Kirtland C. Peterson
Staub-Peterson: Consultation, Training, Development, Inc.
Greensboro, North Carolina

Maurice F. Prout and Robert A. Schwarz
Widener University
Institute for Graduate Clinical Psychology
Chester, Pennsylvania

PLENUM PRESS • NEW YORK AND LONDON

Library of Congress Cataloging-in-Publication Data

Peterson, Kirtland C.
    Post-traumatic stress disorder : a clinician's guide / Kirtland C.
Peterson, Maurice F. Prout, and Robert A. Schwarz.
        p.   cm. -- (The Plenum series on stress and coping)
    Includes bibliographical references and index.
    ISBN 0-306-43542-X
    1. Post-traumatic stress disorder.   I. Prout, Maurice F.
II. Schwarz, Robert A. (Robert Alan), 1956-   . III. Title.
IV. Series.
    [DNLM: 1. Stress Disorders, Post-Traumatic.   WM 170 P485p]
RC552.P67P47   1990
616.85'21--dc20
DNLM/DLC
for Library of Congress   90-14309
                                                               CIP

ISBN 0-306-43542-X

The writers equally share in primary authorship.

© 1991 Plenum Press, New York
A Division of Plenum Publishing Corporation
233 Spring Street, New York, N.Y. 10013

Printed in the United States of America

To Victoria, for her enduring love; and Karl, born in the midst of chaos.

—KCP

To Chris and Jeremy, who have enriched my personal life well beyond the horizon; and to Helen, the best of the long-distance runners.

—MFP

To my wife Kim, and to my family, who have always believed in me.

—RAS

Preface

For hundreds of years, the human response to personal and collective catastrophe has been recognized. Major historical events of the twentieth century have highlighted the reality of the human response to extreme traumatization, especially the experience of persons exposed to the concentration camps of Nazi Germany, the dropping of atomic bombs on Hiroshima and Nagasaki, and the unique features of the Vietnam conflict. However, it was not until 1980, with the publication of the third edition of the *Diagnostic and Statistical Manual* (DSM-III), that post-traumatic stress disorder (PTSD) was fully recognized as a distinct and valid diagnostic category with a permanency not hitherto afforded post-trauma stress syndromes.

Consequently, a formidable PTSD literature has emerged since the late 1970s. Included among the wealth of research and clinical papers are a variety of edited books containing contributions from the major authorities in the field (e.g., Figley, 1978, 1985; van der Kolk, 1984; Kelly, 1985; Sonnenberg, Blank, & Talbott, 1985; Milgram, 1986; Ochberg, 1988). However, to date no publication has brought together and integrated the variety of theoretical and therapeutic perspectives in a form readily accessible to clinicians. It is to this gap in the literature that this contribution is addressed.

Part I deals with the diagnosis and assessment of PTSD. A thorough understanding of the major symptoms and associated features of PTSD, as well as the subtypes and course of the disorder, form the backbone of assessment procedures. Given the many difficulties surrounding the accurate diagnosis of PTSD, appropriate assessment procedures are indicated. The multitude of theoretical explanations for the development of PTSD and subsequent symptomatic picture are presented in Part II. Finally, Part III outlines the various therapeutic modalities that have been used in the treatment of PTSD. A substantial reference list is also provided at the end of the volume.

PTSD is a very real, and serious, clinical syndrome. It appears that the human organism is not biologically programmed to integrate and fully work through massive psychic trauma. There is little doubt that an awareness of PTSD, together with a knowledge of treatment options, will aid clinicians in the assessment and treatment of patients who have experienced repeated childhood incest, rape, violent assault, combat, death camps, natural disasters, kidnapping and hostage situations, bombings, and other forms of extreme traumatization. Indeed, with the increased activity of terrorists worldwide, the horrific possibility of future nuclear accidents, and the threat of nuclear exchanges, the importance of the recognition, evaluation, and treatment of PTSD becomes more crucial with each passing year.

We hope that the data, observations, and suggestions discussed in this work prove helpful to clinicians in the field. The layout of the book, as well as the manner in which various topics are focused and addressed, are designed for easy reference. Although the majority of papers and books about PTSD deal with the experience of the Vietnam combat veteran, we have attempted to make the material presented applicable to all patient populations manifesting PTSD. We hope that greater recognition of the disorder and the specific interventions required for successful resolution will reduce the tremendous pain and suffering felt by those who have undergone extreme traumatization.

Contents

PART I. THE DIAGNOSIS

Chapter 1. History.. 3

Descriptive Aspects 3
Changes in Theoretical Understanding 4
Therapy 6
Cultural and Political Influences............................ 7
Future Trends 8

Chapter 2. Primary Symptoms 11

Introduction 11
Differences between DSM-III and DSM-III-R 12
The Context: The Traumatic Stressor........................ 15
Reexperiencing the Trauma................................. 16
Persistent Avoidance and Numbing of Responsiveness to the
   External World 21
Avoidance Behaviors 25
Increased Arousal... 26
Survivor Guilt and Other Forms of Guilt 31
Summary 34

Chapter 3. Secondary Symptoms 35

Introduction 35
Depression/Dysthymic Disorder 36
Anxiety... 37
Death Imprint/Death Anxiety................................ 37
Impulsive Behavior 38
Substance Abuse.. 38
Somatization/Tension... 39
Alterations in Time Sense.................................... 40
Changes in Ego Functioning 41
Miscellaneous Secondary Features 41
Summary 42

Chapter 4. Subtypes and Course of the Disorder.............. 43

Subtypes.. 43
Course of the Disorder 45
    General Features 46
    Course of the Disorder in Victims of Military Combat 51
    Course of the Disorder in Rape/Assault Victims 51
    Course of the Disorder in Victims of Accidental Man-Made
        Disasters.. 55
    Course of the Disorder in Hiroshima Survivors.............. 58
    Course of the Disorder in Residents of Three Mile Island 59
Summary 60

Chapter 5. PTSD in Children 61

Occurrence.. 61
Symptoms... 62
Parental Responses... 64
    Parental Underreporting.................................. 64
Summary 65

PART II. THEORIES

Chapter 6. Theoretical Perspectives 69

Introduction 69

An Information-Processing Model.......................... 69
A Psychosocial Framework for Understanding the Disorder...... 72
A Behavioral (Learning Theory) Formulation 75
Cognitive Appraisal Models................................ 78
A Psychodynamic ("Classical") Formulation 82
A Psychosocial-Developmental (Erikson)/Psychoformative
    (Lifton) Model.. 84
A Psychoformative Perspective 86
An Object Relations Theory Formulation.................... 88
Psychophysiologic/Psychobiologic Models 91
A Cybernetic Model.. 94
Summary: An Ecosystemic Model 96

PART III. ASSESSMENT

Chapter 7. The Assessment 107

Introduction 107
Formal Diagnostic Procedure for DSM-III-R Diagnosis.......... 108
Structured Interview....................................... 110
Formal Mental Status Examination 111
Psychometric and Psychodiagnostic Testing 111
    Traditional Batteries.................................. 111
    MMPI... 112
    Multimethod Behavioral Assessment 114
    Paper and Pencil Inventories........................... 114
Differential Diagnosis 115
    Anxiety Disorders..................................... 116
    Depressive Disorders.................................. 116
    Adjustment Disorders.................................. 116
    Antisocial Personality Disorders 118
    Schizophrenia... 120
    Factitious PTSD and Malingering 120
Functional Evaluation of the Individual 123
    Pre-Trauma History 124
    Immediate Pre-Trauma Psychosocial Context 124
    The Event and the Immediate Coping Responses........... 124
    Post-Trauma Psychosocial Context 125
    Assessment of Attribution of Meaning................... 126
    Assessing Strengths and Resources...................... 126

Assessment of PTSD in Forensic Situations: Guidelines and
    Methodologies... 127
  Ethical Issues Working for the Defense 127
  Ethical Issues Working for the Plaintiff..................... 128
  An Appropriate Mind-Set for Forensic Evaluations 129
  The Forensic Evaluation of PTSD 129
  Interpretation and Conclusion of the Evaluation............. 132
Problems in Assessment and Diagnosis........................ 133
  Professional Bias 133
  Denial of Diagnosis Workability............................ 134
  Resistance to DSM-III Criteria............................. 134
  Styles of Claimants and Examiners......................... 135
  Lack of Corroboration 136
  The "Silent" Patient....................................... 136
  Exaggeration and Falsification 136
  Intercurrent Stress 137
  "Either-Or" Diagnoses 138
  The Comorbidity Theory................................... 138
  Impact on Examiners 138
Summary 139

PART IV. THERAPY

Chapter 8. General Considerations 143

Introduction 143
Therapy Should Occur Sooner Rather Than Later.............. 143
Therapy Should Be Brief 144
Ego-Supportive Interventions 146
Decreasing Avoidance 146
Normalizing the Abnormal 147
Altering the Attribution of Meaning.......................... 148
Recurring Problems in Treatment 148
Summary 149

Chapter 9. Dynamic Psychotherapy 151

Introduction 151
Theoretical Orientation 151
Procedures... 152
Assessment... 152

General Stratagem of Treatment 154
Goals, Phases, and Priorities of Therapy 155
Treatment of Patients with Hysterical Styles of Information
     Processing.. 156
Treatment of Patients with Obsessional Styles of Information
     Processing.. 157
Effectiveness 158

Chapter 10. Behavioral Treatment 159

Introduction 159
Theoretical Assumptions 159
Implosive Therapy/Imaginal Flooding........................ 160
    Procedure 160
    Effectiveness 162
Systematic Desensitization 163
    Procedure 163
    Effectiveness 164
Behavioral Rehearsal.. 164
Stress Inoculation Training 165
    Effectiveness 169

Chapter 11. Hypnotherapy and Narcosynthesis............... 171

Hypnotherapy.. 171
    Theoretical Assumptions................................ 171
    Hypnotic Procedures 172
    Indications and Contraindications....................... 178
    Effectiveness 179
Narcosynthesis... 180
    Theoretical Assumptions................................ 180
    Indications/Contraindications........................... 180
    Procedure 181
    Effectiveness 181

Chapter 12. Group Treatment 183

Introduction 183
Theoretical Orientations.................................... 183
Procedures 184

Interactively Oriented Group Psychotherapy 184
Cognitive-Behavioral Group Treatment 185
Psychodynamically Oriented Group Psychotherapy 187
Dream Seminars 190
Combined Individual and Group Therapy 191
Effectiveness 191

Chapter 13. Family and Couples Therapy 193

Introduction 193
Theoretical Assumptions 194
Procedures 194
Goals of Family Therapy 194
Characteristics of Post-Traumatic Families 196
Phases of Treatment 198
Treatment Strategies/Goals 201
The Therapist's Role 202
Integration of Family Therapy with Other Modalities 202
Problematic Periods 203
Effectiveness 203

Chapter 14. Therapy of Children with PTSD 205

Introduction 205
Stage 1: Opening 205
Stage 2: Trauma 206
Coping with the Traumatic Experience 207
Stage 3: Closure 208
Summary 212

Chapter 15. Psychopharmacological Treatment 213

Introduction 213
Rationales for Drug Therapy 213
Treatment of Autonomic Arousal and Anxiety 214
Sleep Disturbances 215
Depression 215
Psychotic-like Symptoms 216
Summary 216

Chapter 16. Summary 217

Future Trends 218
Prevention 218
    Prevention Interventions 219
Changes in Theory 219
Changes in Assessment 220
Changes in Therapy 220

Notes 223

References 227

Index 247

I

Diagnosis

1

History

We think it is important to place our current understanding of post-traumatic stress disorder (PTSD) in an historical context. Therefore, we will briefly outline the changes in the concept of traumatic disorders over the last 100 years, as well as the factors that have influenced those changes. Four dimensions of PTSD will be considered:

1. Descriptive aspects
2. Changes in theoretical understanding
3. Therapy
4. Cultural and political influences

DESCRIPTIVE ASPECTS

Trimble (1985) has reported the following changes in the descriptions of PTSD: The term "compensation nerosis" was initiated by Rigler in 1879. This followed an increased rate of invalidism reported after railway accidents, after the introduction of compensation laws in Prussia. The number of claims against the railway companies was so great that the syndrome became known as "railway spine." As a result of the First World War, Mott (1919) coined the term "shell shock." By 1941, Kardiner was using the term "traumatic neurosis."

Interestingly enough, PTSD appears to have led a relatively ignored life as an official diagnostic category. There was not a single mention of any type of trauma related disorder, not even traumatic neurosis or combat neurosis in DSM-I (1952) or DSM-II (1968). In 1980,

PTSD was officially recognized in the DSM-III. The descriptive aspects will be discussed in Chapter 2. In fact, PTSD was the only "neurotic" disorder that had no precursor in the previous DSM's. Finally, the description of PTSD has undergone a few refinements in the DSM-III-R.

CHANGES IN THEORETICAL UNDERSTANDING

Reports of symptoms and syndromes with PTSD-like features have existed in writings throughout the centuries. Trimble (1981) has traced the first theoretical discussion of a post-traumatic syndrome in the medical community to the work of Erichsen, entitled *On the Concussion of the Spine: Nervous Shock and Other Obscure Injuries of the Nervous System in Their Clinical and Medico-Legal Aspects.* The thesis of the work was that relatively mild trauma could cause serious impairment in functioning. The etiology was hypothesized to be neurologic. There ensued a lively debate as to whether or not the condition was neurological or psychological, with a strong side argument for the condition to be one of malingering. Trimble (1985) reported that originally, the etiology of shell shock was thought to be brought about by changes in atmospheric pressure or excess carbon monoxide as a result of battle.

Nevertheless, the psychological formulation gained supremacy. However, there was little elaboration as to the mechanism of the illness (at least with respect to present day standards). At the turn of the century, hysteria became the chief explanatory principle for traumatic reactions. An important shift came with the early analytic writers. They emphasized the significance of "psychological trauma" as opposed to a psychological reaction to a physical trauma. They stressed that it was the overexcitation of the drives of the individual that was traumatic. The overstimulation led to a disturbance of the psychic equilibrium (Fenichel, 1946).

In the early 1900s trauma-related disorders were psychoneuroses of individuals and their drives. The next step involved a decrease in the importance of the drives, and an increased attention given to the ego. Traumatic neurosis was viewed as the ego's inability to master the degree of trauma that resulted in the disorganization of ego-functionining (Kardiner, 1941). At this point the etiology of post-traumatic neurosis is still squarely within the individual.

Trimble(1981) aptly points out that the shift from early analytic writings to later ones represented a shift from the concept of trauma-activating conflicts within the agencies of the mind to the concept of adaptation. Adaptation refers to the attempts of the individual to respond to changes in the environment. Post-traumatic neurosis was seen as a result of failed adaptation. Here we see the first significant movement towards the acknowledgment of the saliency of the ecological demands of reality. It was certainly not a coincidence that these changes took place after the start of World War II. This relationship would be a harbinger of future changes in the understanding of PTSD.

With a few exceptions, virtually nothing was written about post-traumatic neurosis from 1950 to 1970. In the mean time, psychology in general was undergoing many changes. Cognitive and behavioral theories were having increasing influence in the field. Systemic and ecological formulations of pathology and health were also gaining importance. The 1970s and 1980s have seen an explosion in the amount of research and writing on trauma-related disorders. Clearly, the psychological casualties of the Vietnam war were largely responsible for the renewed interest in post-traumatic neurosis. Most of the early papers on post-traumatic neurosis were about Vietnam veterans.

The new emphasis was on the stressors themselves. Eventually, strong empirical support was gathered for the primacy of the traumatic nature of the stressor as the causal agent of PTSD. Even the new name for the disorder, Post-Traumatic *Stress* Disorder, reflected the growing importance of the stressor itself.

Learning theory, particularly the roles of classical conditioning and stimulus generalization became leading explanatory principles for the learned fear response to highly toxic traumas. Instrumental learning was postulated to underlie the avoidance response characteristic of PTSD.

The environmental orientation of behaviorists was further supported by the growing sophistication in the understanding of stressors. The response of "the system" became viewed as a potential source of support or secondary victimization. A supportive response could ameliorate or prevent symptom formation. An unsupportive environment could exacerbate or precipitate symptom development. Even analytic writers (e.g., Horowitz, 1986) gave increased importance to the role of the stressor itself in overloading the individuals capacity to process data.

Finally, the role of cognitive attribution has become a central factor in understanding the dynamics of PTSD. In fact, attribution theory has added a much needed counterbalance to the growing emphasis on the external role of the environmental stressor. Once again, the internal processes of individuals, namely, how they impart meaning to their experiences, are seen as a final common pathway toward the development of PTSD or adaptation. The theoretical role of cognitions in PTSD contains several facets.

First, there is the underlying epistemology of constructivism. Namely, psychological reality is constructed. Since it is constructed, if something happens (i.e., truama) that destroys some of the "girders" of the construction, then repair work must take place. The more devastating the destruction, the more involved the repair work, up to and including the building of an entirely new structure. Out of this view comes the recent recognition that many of the symptoms of PTSD are reflections of the adaptive processes involved in assimilating the new data (i.e., the trauma) and or making accommodations (repairs) in the internal structure of reality (Janoff-Bulman, 1985; Epstein, 1990).

A second facet is the continuation of the analytic emphasis on previous conflicts and personality patterns as being relevant to PTSD. However, a significant shift has occurred. Intrapsychic organization or conflict is not seen as the cause of PTSD. It is viewed as important in understanding the individual variations in symptom presentation. This position is largely supported by the work of cognitively oriented clinicians who also look at the internal individual attributions as central in understanding a specific person's problem.

THERAPY

First, let us summarize Horowitz's (1986) historical review of the treatment strategies for PTSD: Psychological treatment of PTSD became necessary as a result of the combat neuroses that developed in World Wars I and II. The earliest "treatment" was to counteract the fear of injury with a greater threat of real pain. The soldiers with combat neurosis were given excruciating electric shock treatment. Many soldiers did return to the front. Other soldiers committed suicide.

In World War II abreaction and catharsis were used, often using hypnosis and narcohypnosis. The reenactments of traumas were dramatic. However, it was found that it was also important to work through the experience so that the patient understands the meaning of what happened and can revise the negative self-view that often occurs. In addition, it was found to be helpful to include brief periods of rest and recreation. The use of groups was also seen as desirable in order to restore group ties. In regard to combat-related PTSD it was found that treating the soldier as close to the front as possible, and as briefly as posssible, returned the most soldiers to action.

More modern interventions specifically for trauma-related issues have been defined as brief or time-limited. Lindemann's (1944) work on reinstigating the grieving process, and Caplan's (1961) emphasis on viewing periods of crisis as fluid moments with increased possibilities for change, were singled out as important milestones (Horowitz, 1986).

Horowitz's model for time-limited brief dynamic psychotherapy of stress disorders (1976, 1986) places emphasis on matching treatment interventions to phases of the disorder. When the person is in a denial phase, evocative procedures must be used. During intrusive periods when the individual is overwhelmed, supportive and suppressive techniques are used. The goal is to keep the individual in an optimum level of comfort/discomfort for the therapeutic work to continue.

A parallel development in brief interventions has occurred with behavior therapy. Most of the studies have been with Vietnam veterans. Interventions have included systematic desensitization (Kipper, 1977; Schilder, 1980; Mccaffrey & Fairbank, 1985); Implosive therapy (Fairbank & Keane, 1982; Keane et al., 1985); and Behavioral Rehearsal (Fairbank et al., 1981). These interventions are highly focused to the target symptoms. One problem with these studies is that for the most part they are case histories. A second problem is that they only use one type of population. Veronen and Kilpatrick (1983) have successfully used Stress Inoculation Training with large numbers of rape victims.

As recognition of the importance of the ecological niche of the PTSD patient has increased, there has been a rise in the number of reports of family and couples work with PTSD (Figley & Sprenkle, 1978; Jurich, 1983; Danieli, 1985, Figley, 1988). Group settings have been used in psychodynamic modalities (Frick & Bogart, 1982); Cognitive Behavioral approaches (Marafiote, 1980); Hypnotic (Gilligan & Kennedy, in press). As one might expect, there has been a convergence of goals in the treatment of PTSD, despite the different schools of thought.

CULTURAL AND POLITICAL INFLUENCES

At the risk of being inflammatory, we would like to discuss some of the cultural and political issues that have been involved in the diagnosis of PTSD. The central thesis that we would like to raise is that there appears to have been a great deal of resistance to the concept of psychological problems coming from physical trauma. In fact, one of the problems has been the denial that certain traumas even occur. Perhaps the most glaring instance of this phenomenon was Freud's abandonment of the seduction theory (Masson, 1988). Whatever the reason for the abandonment of the seduction theory, it paralleled the de-emphasis on environmental factors in traumatic situations previously discussed.

A related issue can be seen in the socioeconomic stimuli that activate the interest in PTSD. The interest in PTSD occurs after wars, when men are hurt. On the other hand, it has been only very recently (with a few exceptions) that there has been interest in PTSD in rape victims. This is strange for two reasons. First, it is a more common problem than war. More women are raped than men go to war. Second, rape would be a classical trauma for studying PTSD. Nevertheless, there is very little research (with some exceptions) with rape victims.

Another economic problem with respect to PTSD has been the adversarial positions of insurance companies, as well as the legal system. Perhaps it will not surprise the reader to learn that there have been few, if any, fundamental changes in the legal issues involved in PTSD. The players are essentially the same. The plaintiffs are usually individuals who have been in accidents or are veterans. The defendants are usually insurance companies or the government. The central question is always whether or not the person is *really* suffering as a direct result of the trauma, and the extent to which their life has been altered.

While we do not suggest that corporations or the government do not have a right to contain costs, the manner in which these cost-containment procedures are handled sometimes impinges upon the ethics of the psychological profession. For instance, if a clinician evaluates a person for PTSD after an accident and finds significant evidence of accident-related problems, but also finds a small amount of evidence of nonaccident factors, he or she may feel compelled to avoid mentioning the nonaccident factors. The reason is that in many instances, insurance companies will not pay for the evaluation (or treatment) if there is even a hint of other problems. This policy impairs the objectivity of clinicians. The net result is that on a macroscopic level the accurate diagnosis of PTSD may be inhibited.

FUTURE TRENDS

It is likely that there will be a broadening of the contexts in which PTSD will be deemed relevant. Certainly, the experiences of rape and sexual abuse merit inclusion as stressors of sufficiently severe proportions to meet DSM-III-R criteria for trauma. Early childhood hospitalizations may also be relevant contexts for assessing PTSD. There has already been a trend to associate loss, such as through death of a loved one, with PTSD.

This latter context is an area that perhaps best fits another trend that is almost certain to develop in the next few years. Namely, it will be necessary to make sure that the construct of PTSD does not become too broad. There is likely to be an increasing sophistication in the diagnostic distinctions clinicians make. For instance, it is not appropriate to say that the death of an 80-year-old father is a stressor beyond the realm of normal human experience.[1] However, the loss of a 5-year-old child may be considered beyond normal expectations.

Economic and political forces will remain strong influences in the field of PTSD. The increased sophistication of technology appears to lead to increasingly more elaborate disasters (e.g., Three Mile Island and Chernobyl). Under the Reagan administration there was an attitude of lassitude with regard to environmental protection, as well as safety in the workplace. It is quite probable that these factors will result in more accidents, and therefore, more diagnoses of PTSD. As PTSD becomes a more accepted diagnosis, it is probable that it will be used more often in legal battles. As a result, two opposing trends may occur. One will be increased entrenchment on the part of insurance companies to limit payments by denying the existence or relevance of psychological factors in accidents (work-related or otherwise). The other possibility will be a realization that denying the problem does not make it go away. In this more progressive approach, primary and secondary prevention methods will be utilized to cut costs. It certainly may be necessary for clinical researchers to demonstrate the cost-effectiveness of early intervention for PTSD.

In the area of therapy, it is hoped that there will be more research using better methodology. Although there is no evidence to support this claim, we would like to suggest that PTSD is an excellent diagnostic entity to use for psychotherapy research.

2

Primary Symptoms

INTRODUCTION

An understanding of the diagnostic criteria for PTSD is crucial for a thorough assessment of the disorder. To this effect a substantial proportion of the literature is concerned directly or indirectly with the symptomatic picture of patients with PTSD.

In this presentation of the clinical characteristics of PTSD a distinction has been made between "primary" and "secondary" symptoms. Primary symptoms are those which form the basis for the diagnostic criteria of PTSD according to the DSM-III and DSM-III-R. These are noted in Tables 2.1 and 2.2. A discussion of these symptoms is the focus of this chapter. The primary symptoms as outlined in the DSM-III and DSM-III-R are supplemented with the wealth of data in the literature directly addressing these clinical phenomena. Greater awareness of the nature of the central-symptom clusters aids in the assessment and positive diagnosis of PTSD. Although much of the literature is devoted to Vietnam combat veterans, many of the clinical observations are readily generalized to other patient populations with PTSD.

Secondary symptoms (or "associated features") of PTSD refer to symptoms and symptom clusters which commonly coexist with PTSD, but do not form part of the diagnostic criteria for the disorder. They are part of the larger, and more complex, clinical picture presented by PTSD patients. Secondary symptoms are the subject of Chapter 3.

Table 2.1. Diagnostic Criteria for Post-Traumatic Stress Disorder (DSM-III, 1980)

A. Existence of a recognizable stressor that would evoke significant symptoms of distress in almost everyone

B. Reexperiencing of the trauma as evidenced by at least one of the following:
   (1) recurrent and intrusive recollections of the event
   (2) recurrent dreams of the event
   (3) sudden acting or feeling as if the traumatic event were recurring, because of an association with an environmental or ideational stimulus

C. Numbing or responsiveness to or reduced involvement with the external world, beginning some time after the trauma, as shown by at least one of the following:
   (1) markedly diminished interest in one or more significant activities
   (2) feeling of detachment or estrangement from others
   (3) constricted affect

D. At least two of the following symptoms that were not present before the trauma:
   (1) hyperalertness or exaggerated startle response
   (2) sleep disturbance
   (3) guilt about surviving while others have not, or about behavior required for survival
   (4) memory impairment or trouble concentrating
   (5) avoidance of activities that arouse recollection of the traumatic event
   (6) intensification of symptoms by exposure to events that symbolize or resemble the traumatic event

DIFFERENCES BETWEEN DSM-III AND DSM-III-R

While the essential features of PTSD remain the same in the DSM-III and DSM-III-R, there are several important differences. The most important change is an increased emphasis on avoidance in the DSM-III-R. This cluster of symptoms has been associated with the numbing of general responsiveness symptoms. The criteria for avoidance are listed under section C. They include:

1. Efforts to avoid thoughts or feelings associated with trauma.
2. Efforts to avoid activities or situations that arouse recollections of the trauma.
3. Inability to recall an important aspect of the trauma. (p. 250)

One of the reasons the committee included these criteria is that they are easily operationalized from a behavioral perspective, unlike psychic numbing (Keane, personal communication, February 18, 1988). In addition, the elaboration of these avoidance-based symptoms reflects an appreciation of the importance of these phenomena in the diagnosis of PTSD, their relevance in the promulgation of PTSD, and their significance in its treatment.

There is increasing evidence that avoidance of painful material is a

Table 2.2. Diagnostic Criteria for Post-Traumatic Stress Disorder (DSM-III-R, 1987)

A. The individual has experienced an event that is outside the range of usual human experience and that would be markedly distressing to almost anyone, e.g., serious threat to one's life or physical integrity; serious threat or harm to one's children, spouse, or other close relatives or friends; sudden destruction of one's home or community; or seeing another person who has been, is being (or has recently been), seriously injured or killed as the result of an accident or physical violence.

B. The traumatic event is persistently reexperienced in at least one of the following ways:
   (1) recurrent and intrusive distressing recollections of the event (in young children, repetitive play in which themes or aspects of the trauma are expressed)
   (2) recurrent distressing dreams of the event
   (3) sudden acting or feeling as if the traumatic event were recurring (includes a sense of reliving the experience, illusions, hallucinations, and dissociative [flashback] episodes, even those that occur upon waking or when intoxicated)
   (4) intense psychological distress at exposure to events that symbolize or resemble an aspect of the traumatic event, including anniversaries of trauma

C. Persistent avoidance of stimuli associated with the trauma or numbing of general responsiveness (not present before the trauma), as indicated by at least three of the following:
   (1) deliberate efforts to avoid thoughts or feelings associated with the trauma
   (2) deliberate efforts to avoid activities or situations that arouse recollections of the trauma
   (3) inability to recall an important aspect of the trauma (psyhogenic amnesia)
   (4) markedly diminished interest in significant activities (in young children, loss of recently acquired developmental skills such as toilet training or language skills)
   (5) feeling of detachment or estrangement from others
   (6) restricted range of affect, e.g., unable to have loving feelings
   (7) sense of foreshortened future, e.g., child does not expect to have a career, marriage, or children, or a long life

D. Persistent symptoms of increased arousal (not present before the trauma) as indicated by at least two of the following:
   (1) difficulty falling or staying asleep
   (2) irritability or outbursts of anger
   (3) difficulty concentrating
   (4) hypervigilance
   (5) exaggerated startle response
   (6) physiologic reactivity at exposure to events that symbolize or resemble an aspect of the traumatic event (e.g., a woman who was raped in an elevator breaks out in a sweat when entering any elevator)

E. Duration of the disturbance of at least one month. Specify delayed onset if the onset of symptoms was at least six months after the trauma.

central mechanism in PTSD. Malloy et al.(1983) found that the single best predictor of the diagnosis of PTSD in Vietnam veterans was the strong tendency of veterans with PTSD to terminate the viewing of simulated reenactments of combat material. One of the central principles for treatment across schools of thought (e.g. behavioral, psycho-dynamic, hypnotic) is to allow the patient to face (stop avoiding) the painful material in a manner that allows for extinction or mastery of the trauma.

The second difference between DSM-III and DSM-III-R is an elaboration of the syndrome in children. The new paragraphs in DSM-III-R read:

> **Age-specific factors.** Occasionally, a child may be mute or refuse to discuss the trauma, but this should not be confused with inability to remember what occurred. In younger children, distressing dreams of the event may, within several weeks, change into generalized nightmares of monsters, of rescuing others, or of threats to self or others. Young children do not have the sense that they are reliving the past; reliving the trauma occurs in action through repetitive play.
>
> Diminished interest in significant activities and constrictions of affect both may be difficult for children to report on themselves, and should be carefully evaluated by reports from parents, teachers, and other observers. A symptom of Post-traumatic Stress Disorder in children may be foreshortened future; for example, a child may not expect to have a career or marriage. There may also be "omen formation," that is, belief in an ability to prophesy future untoward events.
>
> Children may exhibit various physical symptoms, such as stomachaches and headaches, in addition to the specific symptoms of increased arousal noted above. (APA, 1987 p. 249)

The new description for symptoms in children includes:

> B. (1) recurrent and intrusive distressing recollections of the event (*in young children, repetitive play in which themes or aspects of the trauma are expressed*)
>
> C. (4) markedly diminished interest in significant activities (*in young children loss of recently acquired developmental skills such as toilet training or language skills*) (p. 250)

The third change involved in the DSM-III-R was the removal of "survivor guilt"[2] from the criteria list. It was dropped to an associated feature. The rationale has been recounted by Keane (1988).

1. The committee felt that the symptom of "survivor guilt" was, in fact, unique to PTSD.
2. However, it did not appear to be general enough to cover the many different types of guilt associated with PTSD. Therefore, survivor guilt was expanded to guilt in general.
3. Unfortunately, the rules for classification of a disorder in the DSM-III-R include the procedure to use as few symptoms as necessary to differentiate one disorder from another. The problem became that guilt in general did not differentiate PTSD from other disorders, such as depression. Therefore, guilt and survivor guilt were delegated to the category of associated features.

Finally, the inclusion of the avoidance symptoms as well as the increased detail of criteria related to exposure to symbolic representation of the traumatic event [See criteria B. (4), which is completely new, and D. (6)] indicates an increased appreciation of the importance of symbolic representation in the cognitive views of PTSD. It also reflects a more sophisticated elaboration of the roles of generalization gradients of anxiety.

THE CONTEXT: THE TRAUMATIC STRESSOR

The most crucial aspect of the PTSD diagnosis is establishing the nature of the traumatic stressor.

Although various critics of the PTSD diagnosis have criticized the lack of refinement of the concept of "traumatic stressor" (Figley, 1985), various guidelines have been put forward. As outlined in the DSM-III and DSM-III-R criteria, the stressor must be (1) psychologically distressing; (2) markedly distressing to almost anyone; and (3) outside the range of "usual human experience."

Examples of such events help to further refine the concept. The most common categories of traumatic stressors that lead to PTSD include rape, violent assault, military combat, natural disasters (e.g., floods, earthquakes, tornadoes, etc.), accidental disasters (e.g., car accidents with serious physical injury, airplane crashes, large fires, collapse of physical structures, accidents at sea, etc.), man-made disasters (e.g., bombing, torture, death camps, hostage taking, terrorism, etc.)(American Psychiatric Association, 1980, 1987).

The essential characteristics of traumatic events include (but are not restricted to) (1) a serious threat to one's life; (2) a serious threat to one's physical integrity; (3) a serious threat or possible harm to one's children/spouse/close relative/friends; (4) sudden destruction of one's home/community; (5) seeing another person who has been/is being/has recently been seriously injured or killed; (6) physical violence; and (7) learning about serious threat/harm to relative/family.

Often the traumatic event includes a physical component, usually direct damage to the central nervous system. Examples include head injuries and malnutrition (American Psychiatric Association, 1980; 1987).

In addition to the criteria outlined in the DSM-III and DSM-III-R, the literature on PTSD has referred to the "traumatic stressor" with reference to a variety of significant catastrophes and traumatic events. These include the concentration camps of Nazi Germany, the experience of combat troops in Vietnam, the Hyatt Regency Hotel disaster, the Buffalo Creek catastrophe, the Hills and Coconut Grove fires, violent rape and/or assault, the bombing of Hiroshima and Nagasaki, and so on.

REEXPERIENCING THE TRAUMA

Intrusive Thoughts, Feelings, Images, Memories. The element of reexperiencing the traumatic event is a salient aspect of PTSD (Horowitz, 1974; 1976; Horowitz et al., 1980). Reexperiencing the trauma takes a number of forms. For positive diagnosis of PTSD only one form of reexperiencing the original stressor need be present.

Recurrent/Distressing Disturbing Recollections of Event. The most common form of intrusion is involuntary recollection of the stressor. Thoughts, feelings, images, and memories of the traumatic event emerge into conscious awareness and are experienced as disturbing to the patient. Attempts to suppress this material are frequently difficult, if not impossible. Intrusions, when present in this form, are a recurring feature of the clinical picture.

Aspects of the event, or of the patient's reactions to the event, were repeated in these recollections. Most frequently these included (1) pangs of emotion, (2) rumination or preoccupation, (3) fear of losing bodily control, (4) fear of hyperactivity in any bodily system, (5) intrusive ideas in word form, (6) difficulty dispelling ideas, and (7) intrusive images (Horowitz et al., 1980).

Horowitz et al. (1980) in their study of patients with stress-response syndromes, note that intrusive ideas and feelings were present in 75% of the population studied. Krupnick and Horowitz (1981) isolate 10 common themes manifested in intrusive thoughts:

- rage at source (of the serious life event)
- sadness over loss
- discomfort over (discovered personal) vulnerability
- discomfort over (reactive) aggressive impulses
- fear of loss of control over aggressive impulses
- guilt over responsibility (for inciting the event of failing to prevent it)
- fear of similarity to victim
- rage at those exempted (from loss or injury)
- fear of repetition (of the event)
- survivor guilt

To the above themes Goodwin (1980) adds the replaying of problematical aspects of traumas, including the search for alternative out-comes to the event. Kinzie (1986) reports that over 75% of Cambodian refugees with PTSD reported recurrent and intrusive thoughts. Wilkin-son (1983), in his study of survivors of the Hyatt Regency Hotel disaster, reports repeated recollections of the event in over 85% of subjects ques-tioned. Recollections of the original trauma are also commonly found in other patient populations manifesting PTSD.

Intrusive thoughts, affects, images, and memories are experienced as uncomfortable by patients. Wilmer (1982c) notes that these intrusive recollections may lead to fear, panic, or possible violent acting out in Vietnam combat veterans. Krupnick (1980) echoes this concern with victims of violent crimes.

Recurrent Distressing Dreams/Nightmares. Repetitive dreams and nightmares are another common way in which intrusive thoughts, feel-ings, images, and memories are reexperienced. Usually the dreams re-peat the event or aspects of the event exactly as they occurred. However, elaborations of the original material are also not uncommon. Wilmer (1982c) notes four categories of nightmare found in patients manifest-ing PTSD symptomatology:

- a recurring nightmare that recapitulates a real experience
- a nightmare of events that were untrue in the dreamer's experi-ence, but that could have happened
- a nightmare of events that were untrue of the original experience, and also improbable (but not impossible)
- a nightmare completely divorced from reality

To diagnose PTSD, dreams and nightmares must present the origi-nal trauma unaltered. Wilmer (1982c) notes that the first category ac-counts for about 45% of reported dreams. Common themes in the dreams of Vietnam veterans include (DeFazio, 1978; Goodwin, 1980):

- being helpless in the face of an attack
- finding oneself alone in a potentially fatal situation
- facing danger with a weapon that will not fire
- getting shot
- being pursued by the enemy
- finding oneself without a weapon

Most frequently these themes are part of traumatic nocturnal reen-actments of the traumatic event, or are intertwined within general dreams about Vietnam.

Horowitz et al. (1980) report that about 50% of patients with stress response syndromes report bad dreams. This finding is confirmed by Wilkinson (1983). Krystal and Niederland (1968) note that over 70% of concentration camp survivors report anxiety dreams and nightmares, and that approximately 40% report severe nightmares. Kinzie (1986) reports that over 75% of the Cambodian refugees with PTSD studied manifested recurrent nightmares. Krupnick (1980) also reports nightmares in victims of violent crimes.

Van der Kolk et al. (1984) found that combat veterans with PTSD tended to have their dreams earlier in the sleep cycle than is common, and had a higher frequency of nightmares. These dreams contained exact replicas of traumatic events and sometimes prompted gross body movements (characteristic of night terrors/stage IV sleep). They also reported that it was possible to differentiate veterans with nightmares subsequent to extreme traumatization from men with a chronic history of nightmares. The latter group tended to manifest thought disorder on psychological testing and had nightmares not dissimilar to their day-time concerns.

Many authors have noted that the dreams and nightmares of PTSD patients often "continue upon waking" (Krystal & Niederland, 1968; Hendin et al., 1984; Blank, 1985b). This is addressed at greater length below in the discussion of dissociative phenomena. Dreams and night-mares recapitulating the original stressor may continue for years, even decades after the event.

Reliving the Event, Illusions, Hallucinations, Flashbacks. Dissociative reactions to extreme traumatization are a less frequently occurring form of intrusion. They have been noted primarily in survivors of concentration camps and combat veterans (populations that have usually experienced multiple traumatic stressors). Hendin et al. (1984) note that flashbacks are more common among Vietnam combat veterans than veterans of World Wars I and II. Blank (1985b) notes certain characteristics commonly found with flashbacks:

- powerful emotions are expressed
- sudden onset
- discontinuity with normal behavior
- post-flashback amnesia/confusion
- direct link to traumatic event(s)
- the "primal nature" of the psychological issues
  (e.g., annihilation vs. nonannihilation)

Duration of dissociative-like states is reported to be from a few minutes to several days in the DSM-III and DSM-III-R descriptions of the disorder. Hendin et al. (1984) add that such phenomena may even persist for years.

Jaffe (1968) has described "quasi-psychotic attacks" and "pseudohallucinatory dissociated states" in survivors of death camps. Niederland (1968) describes chronic "psychosis-like pictures" characterized by nighttime persecutory hallucinations, states of depersonalization, paranoid manifestations, and episodic "hallucinatory or semi-hallucinatory reliving of the past." With reference to the phenomenology of flashbacks in Vietnam combat veterans Hendin et al. (1984) note:

> In reliving experiences the individual is awake but appears to be in a state of altered consciousness and often has subsequent amnesia for what takes place. The experiences last from a few minutes to several hours and can usually be distinguished from startle reactions in response to environmental stimuli that momentarily reinvoke traumatic combat events, in which misperceptions are quickly corrected. (p. 165)

What distinguishes the type of flashback noted above from dissociative phenomena seen in fugues and/or multiple personalities is that Vietnam combat veterans rarely assume the identity of another person during episodes (Hendin et al., 1984).

Blank (1985) goes further than Hendin et al. (1984) and differentiates three distinct forms of revivification:

- vivid dreams followed by waking and the inability to dispell the sense that the dream was real; motoric activity associated with the content of the dream may occur.
- "conscious flashback experiences" involving intrusive, vivid images with the patient not necessarily losing touch with reality; dramatic motor behavior may result; pseudo-hallucinations are common; after the flashback the patient can separate the images from reality.
- "unconscious flashbacks" involving motoric action stimulated by memories, affects, and impulses related to the event, but consciousness is bypassed (manifest psychic content may appear unrelated or only indirectly related); frequently this kind of flashback is overlooked.

In addition to a variety of external cues, various psychological/physiological states may trigger dissociative phenomena in patients prone to them. These include: insomnia, mental and/or physical fatigue, increased stress, and substance abuse.

In sum, dissociative phenomena are a more dramatic and serious manifestation of the intrusion of thoughts, affect, images, and memories. They appear to be more highly correlated with experiences of multiple traumas (e.g., the experience of combat soldiers in the Vietnam war, the extreme traumatization of the concentration camps, etc.). Dissociative states frequently lead to fear, panic and a loss of control.

Distress at Exposure to Event Symbolizing/Resembling Trauma. Whereas the intensification of symptoms following exposure to events symbolizing or resembling the original traumatic event were included in the "miscellaneous" list of symptoms in the DSM-III, the DSM-III-R grouping of symptoms includes this symptom with other intrusive phenomena.

> Specifically, symptoms characteristic of Post-traumatic Stress Disorder are often intensified when the individual is exposed to situations or activities that resemble or symbolize the original trauma (e.g., cold snowy weather or uniformed guards for death-camp survivors, hot humid weather for veterans of the South Pacific). (American Psychiatric Association, 1980, p. 237)

With reference to Vietnam veterans, Goodwin (1980) stresses that everyday stimuli may remind the veteran of the war zone:

> Many [intrusive] episodes are triggered by common everyday experiences that remind the veteran of the war zone: helicopters flying overhead, the smell of urine (corpses have no muscle tone, and the bladder evacuates at the moment of death), the smell of diesel fuel (the commodes and latrines were filled with diesel fuel and were burned when filled with human excrement), green tree lines (these were searched for any irregularity which often meant the presence of enemy movement), the sound of popcorn popping (the sound is very close to that of small arms fire in the distance), and loud discharge, a rainy day (it rains for months during the monsoons in Vietnam), and finally the sight of Vietnamese refugees. (p. 16)

External cues may prompt various forms of intrusive recall ranging from distressing recollections and increased nightmares to flashbacks and dissociative phenomena.

Following the Hyatt Regency Hotel disaster, approximately 35% of survivors interviewed reported reactiveness to events similar to, or evoking, the original catastrophe (Wilkinson, 1983). Over 50% of the Cambodian refugees with PTSD reported an intensification of symptoms when exposed to events resembling or symbolizing their ordeal. In addition to physical events that evoke the traumatic event, anniversaries may also be a sufficient trigger for intrusive thoughts, affects, imagery, and memories (DSM-III-R description).

It is not surprising that one of the cardinal symptoms of PTSD is the reexperiencing of the trauma. Epstein (1990) has proposed that the reexperiencing of the trauma, while not comfortable, can have adaptive value. Trauma by its very nature is overwhelming. The individual is forced to reexamine the event(s) many times in order to master the experience. Alternative behaviors, assumptions, and beliefs can be considered for adaptive value. Trauma by its very nature is also threatening. A generalization gradient of anxiety in response to cues can provide an early warning psystem that alerts the individual to potential danger. The intrusion of dysphoric material about the trauma can act as a powerful motivator for change, whereas an optimistic and self-confident stance may inhibit effective coping (Wortman, 1983).

In other words, the phenomenon of intrusive ideation and affect after trauma is not, in and of itself, pathological. For various reasons (that will be elucidated later), the ratio of the intensity of the noxiousness to coping ability for some individuals is sufficiently disparate so that the person attempts to avoid the dysphoric material.

It is the attempt to avoid the noxiousness of re-experiencing the trauma or the anxiety of confronting and rebuilding shattered assumptions, (Janoff-Bullman, 1985) that leads to a pathological resolution. In attempting to avoid the painful memories, feelings, and associations, the individual fails to "learn the lesson" that would bring about an adaptive resolution. Healthy resolution is not determined by the cessation of intrusive material. Rather, healthy resolution is more often achieved by using the intrusive material. The more individuals express their feelings about what happened to them, and the more they can find meaning in what happened, the more likely there will be an adaptive outcome (Silver & Wortman, 1980). The intrusive memories and feelings tend to stop when there is little left to be learned and the individuals are wiser but perhaps sadder (Epstein, 1990).

In many instances, it is not the problem that is pathological; rather, it is the attempted solution that causes dysfunction (Weakland et al., 1984). For instance, when a person has an episode of intrusive material, their attempted solution may be to tell themselves how stupid or crazy they must be; and they had better knock it off. More often than not this stance is impossible to achieve. As the person fails at achieving the goal they have set for themselves, further self-criticism ensues with increasing degradation of self-esteem.

PERSISTENT AVOIDANCE AND NUMBING OF RESPONSIVENESS TO THE EXTERNAL WORLD

The second major clinical feature of PTSD is "psychic numbing" (Lifton, 1967), "denial and numbing" (Horowitz, 1974, 1976), or "emotional anesthesia" (Shatan, 1973, 1978; American Psychiatric Association, 1980). The observed numbing of general responsiveness stands in contradistinction to the patient's characteristic responsiveness prior to the trauma (DSM-III-R description). Usually psychic numbing begins shortly after exposure to extreme traumatization (Wilmer, 1982c). Horowitz et al. (1980) found over 65% of patients with stress response syndromes reported numbness and reduced levels of feeling responses to external stimuli.

Diminished Interest in Significant Activities. A common finding among patients manifesting PTSD symptomatology is a loss of interest in activities that previously engaged them (Wilmer, 1982c). In children this often takes the form of the loss of recently acquired developmental skills (e.g., toilet training, language skills, etc.) (DSM-III-R criteria). Withdrawal from social life is part of the clinical syndrome observed in concentration camp survivors (Krystal & Niederland, 1968).

Restricted Range of Affect. Following a traumatic event a person's range of affect often becomes restricted (Lifton, 1976, 1982; Penk et al., 1981). Commonly the person may report loss of feelings associated with intimacy, tenderness, and sexuality. In the most extreme cases a person may lose the capacity to feel any emotions at all (Wilmer, 1982c).

Lifton (1967) discusses the necessity of "psychic closing off" for those who survived the atomic explosions in Japan during World War II, and for those who endured the concentration camps of Nazi Germany. Niederland (1968) notes with respect to the survivors of the death camps:

> All feelings ceased to be, at least on the surface, because one could not exist and at the same time live with such feelings of abhorrence, disgust, and terror. Simultaneous with the isolation of affects, there was an automatization of the ego which produced a robotlike numbness, giving the inmates a sordid-looking, emaciated, puppetlike appearance. (p. 67)

Shatan (1978) notes that with Vietnam veterans, pre-combat training often encouraged psychic numbing (i.e., sensitivity and compassion were inhibited or repressed). Consequently, violent traumas experienced during the war became superimposed on top of an already existing predilection for psychic numbing. The result was marked levels of unresponsiveness to affective stimuli.

Goodwin (1980) notes that the spouses of Vietnam veterans often describe them as cold, unfeeling, and uncaring. Sometimes they are referred to as "emotionally dead" (Shatan, 1973). It has been suggested that the "thawing" of frozen emotions would confront the veteran with memories of extreme traumatization (Goodwin, 1980). Consequently, inner peace is gained through the maintenance of a "dead space" within. Shatan (1978) has described this as a retreat to "mental foxholes."

A phenomenon associated with restriction of affect is the fact that in some PTSD patient populations, especially concentration camp survivors and Vietnam veterans, normal grief and mourning reactions were inhibited. Howard (1976) and Goodwin (1980) note that grief in the field of combat was either impossible or handled in an unrealistically short amount of time. Shatan (1973, 1978) refers to the resulting condition as one of "impacted grief."

Feelings of Detachment/Estrangement. Not infrequently PTSD patients report feelings of detachment and estrangement (American Psychiatric Association, 1980; Wilmer, 1982c). This is commonly manifested in the disrupted family life of the patient and is highly correlated with the restricted range of affect noted above. Roberts et al. (1982) note significant problems in the areas of intimacy and sociability in Vietnam combat veterans not due to premilitary adjustment or confounding demographic variables. Goodwin (1980) notes that Vietnam veterans who have become numb are often troubled by descriptions from family and friends that they are cold, and consequently feel alienated. Detachment or estrangement from others was found in over 50% of Cambodian refugees with PTSD studied by Kinzie (1986).

Penk et al. (1981) note six interpersonal areas in which Vietnam combat troops are likely to have difficulties: (1) getting on with people; (2) getting emotionally close to someone; (3) family problems; (4) marital problems; (5) inability to express feelings to those they care about; and (6) sexual problems.

As noted earlier, these tend to promote feelings of estrangement and detachment. Penk et al. (1981) note that the more extensive the combat experience, the more likely that these areas have been negatively affected.

The feelings of estrangement may be intrapsychicaly determined or may be a result of actual failures of the victim's environment to be supportive. The sequelae of extreme trauma often include the survivors and victims being ignored, actively avoided and devalued. Frequently family and friends are frightened and do not wish to hear about a disaster. With respect to the experience of rape victims, Vietnam combat veterans, and survivors of the holocaust, family, friends, communities, and society as a whole often do not encourage either discussion of these events or reintegration.

Ayalon (1983) reports how Israeli communities often refuse to recognize the special needs of survivors of terrorist attacks, such as demanding that victimized children behave like all the other children or not be so afraid. She also reports that often families of murdered, or more seriously injured victims, express their hostility to survivors.

On the other hand, it is not infrequent that health professionals and support systems inappropriately expect a lack of positive emotion from individuals who have suffered irrevocable loss or victimization (Wortman & Silver, 1987). Sometimes they may actually exert social pressure to express distress and grief, viewing failure to do so as pathological (Ayalon, 1983; Wortman & Silver, 1987). For instance, children who were part of terrorist incidents were expected to *not* laugh and play. It was deemed wrong in light of all the other children who were killed or maimed (Ayalon, 1983). The social demand on survivors to feel and behave in manners not congruent with their inner experience may contribute to their sense of estrangement from others.

DeFazio (1978) and Goodwin (1980) describe well the pressures on returning Vietnam troops, especially the negative labels attached to them (e.g., "psychopathic killer"). Lack of support is also noted. Wilmer (1982c) notes a "withdrawal into painful introverted isolation" with a resulting "nebulous touch between people." Goodwin (1980) notes that feelings of detachment, estrangement, and isolation are also manifested in a constant search for a "safe place" with frequent moving about the country.

Psychogenic Amnesia. The inability to recall certain aspects of the traumatic event is a diagnostic feature that was introduced in the DSM-III-R criteria for PTSD.

Sense of a foreshortened future. This feature is specific to children who have been exposed to extreme traumatization. It describes the phenomenon among children who no longer entertain the normal expectations for the future. Alterations in future expectations include (Terr, 1983a) (1) Philosophical pessimism (the future seen as greatly limited); (2) an unusually short life span; (3) a future disaster; (4) inability to envisage marriage, children; and (5) no occupation.

The future is spoken of with "little confidence and scant hope." Terr (1983a) regards the sense of a foreshortened future as a "temporal perspective disorder." It appears to be the long-term end point of several effects of trauma (Terr, 1983a, 1983b):

- the sense of foreboding and bad luck that are frequently associated with time distortions
- long-standing fears, everyday stimuli (that would not ordinarily cause anxiety)
- the loss of trust

- the experience of personal vulnerability
- the anticipation/fear of future catastrophes
- dreams of personal death

As with psychogenic amnesia this symptom was first introduced in the DSM-III-R criteria.

AVOIDANCE BEHAVIORS

In DSM-III avoidance behaviors were considered a separate group of phenomenon from the central features of PTSD. The new criteria included in the DSM-III-R grouped with the numbing of responsiveness are:

1. efforts to avoid thoughts or feelings associated with trauma
2. efforts to avoid activities or situations that arouse recollections of the trauma
3. inability to recall an important aspect of the trauma. (p. 250)

It seems more accurate to place the numbing of responsiveness as a concomitant of avoidance mechanisms. In the attempt to avoid painful material, the person gradually numbs increasing amounts of emotional material. The paradigm that seems most applicable is the one proposed by Dollard and Miller (1950) for learned repression. It is interesting to note that the example that Dollard and Miller use is combat related. They explain learned repression as follows:

1. During combat the soldier is being stimulated by many external cues and internal cues, such as feelings, thoughts and attributions.
2. The traumatic conditions in combat attach strong fears to *all these* cues. These fears generalize to other similar cues. The stronger the fears are the wider they generalize.
3. Later, when the soldier starts to think about what happened, his thoughts and images are cues that evoke extreme fear.
4. When the soldier stops thinking about the experience, the cues are removed, and the fear diminishes.
5. The reduction in the fear strongly reinforces the response of stopping thinking.
6. "The milder cases lose a relatively few memories...in the most extreme cases all responses of thought, perception and speech stop." (p. 202)

"Psychic numbing" can be viewed as the end product of a generalized avoidance response to an increasing spectrum of internal cues. First, the patient attempts to avoid thoughts, images and feelings directly related to the trauma (first-order association). However, a different thought or feeling reminds the patient of the first order association (second-order association). So, it too is avoided. The process continues until the patient's anxiety is brought under control.

In this paradigm, a man might be numb to the love of his wife, because if there were no repression or avoidance, his associations would run, "I feel so wonderful with my wife.... my body feels so warm and good...this is the best feeling my body has ever had...I have experienced worse feelings...when I was in (Vietnam, Aushwitz, Buffalo Creek...).... A parallel train of thought could be, "I love my wife so much...I am the luckiest man in the world...unlike my best friend who had his legs blown off during the war...."

The nonvolitional aspect of psychic numbing stands in contradistinction to the more conscious behavioral avoidance outlined in DSM-III-R. These behaviors are essentially escape behaviors, motivated and reinforced by the avoidance of anxiety.

INCREASED AROUSAL

Observations of increased physiological and autonomic arousal have frequently been reported in patients who have experienced extreme traumatization. Whereas persistent symptoms of increased arousal were included in the "miscellaneous" grouping of symptoms in the DSM-III, the DSM-III-R criteria place them under one heading. Studies of PTSD Vietnam veterans have demonstrated tonic levels of increased arousal as measured by heart rate (HR) (Malloy, Fairbank, & Keane, 1983; Pallmeyer, Blanchard, & Kolb, 1986) and systolic blood pressure (Pallmeyer et al., 1986).

When presented with visual scenes and auditory sounds or just auditory sounds of war, clinically noticeable (93 bpm to 104 bpm) and statistically significant increases in heart rate have been documented by Malloy, et al. (1983) and Pallmeyer (1986), respectively. Both studies pointed to heart rate as the most robust measure, even though there were statistical differences between PTSD and non-PTSD groups on other measures such as blood pressure and skin response. Using discriminant analyses, both studies could accurately identify PTSD and non-PTSD veterans with accuracies ranging from 80–86%.

In the Malloy et al. study (1983) none of the control groups elected to terminate the presentation of the videotaped scenes; however 8 of 10

PTSD subjects did escape the scenes. The remaining two subjects wept continuously through the scenes. The inclusion of this behavioral measure improved the classification rate to 100%.

Pallmeyer et al. (1986) compared changes of heart rate for the individual subjects across trials. Their rationale was that if HR response is to be used as a diagnostic marker for PTSD, it would need to discriminate patients with PTSD from those with a different disorder at the individual level. They compared the HR response to mental arithmetic to the HR response to an audiotape of combat sounds. They found they accurately diagnosed 83% of the PTSD veterans and 89% of the other subjects when they used a cutoff score of the HR response to combat sounds greater than or equal to 3.5bpm below the noncombat stressor. In other words, non-PTSD subjects were generally much more stressed by the arithmetic problems. PTSD subjects were either much more stressed by the combat sounds or about equally stressed by the two stimuli.

Sleep Difficulties. Sleep disturbances, both dependent and independent of nightmares, are commonly found in PTSD patient populations. Indeed, Krystal and Niederland (1968) report sleep disturbances in nearly 100% of concentration-camp survivors interviewed. DeFazio (1978) refers to sleep difficulties as the "hallmark of reaction to traumatic experience." With respect to Vietnam veterans he notes: "It is almost axiomatic that regardless of how successful a veteran has been in escaping other symptoms, the trauma will tend to be reflected in his dreams and attendant sleep difficulties" (p. 36). Frequently dreams produce a fitful sleep, the veteran often awaking in a cold sweat, sometimes crying out. Penk et al. (1981) note significant differences in sleep difficulties between combat and noncombat troops, as well as between heavy and light combat veterans.

Lavie et al. (1979) note various alterations in the sleep patterns of soldiers who experienced traumatization during the Yom Kippur War. These include (1) significantly longer sleep latencies; (2) lower sleep efficiency indices; (3) lower percentage of REM sleep; and (4) longer REM latencies. The types of sleep difficulties noted included (1) sleep-onset insomnia; (2) nocturnal myoclonus (involuntary muscle twitching during sleep); (3) dream-interruption insomnia; (4) pseudoinsomnia; and (5) nonrestorative sleep syndrome.

Lavie et al. (1979) report that traumatic events have a long-term effect on sleep, often persisting for years. Changes in "sleep architecture" may continue even after the patient has stopped having repetitive nightmares of the traumatic event.

Memory Impairment/Difficulties Concentrating. Three cognitive changes are commonly found in patients with PTSD (American Psychiatric Association, 1980; Wilmer, 1982c). These are (1) impaired memory; (2) concentration difficulties; and (3) difficulties associated with finishing a task.

In confirmation of the above, Horowitz et al. (1980) note that over 75% of patients with stress response syndromes in their study manifested: (1) Trouble concentrating; (2) difficulties making decisions; and (3) trouble remembering things. Over 50% reported having to check/recheck actions taken or performing tasks slowly to insure correctness.

A smaller percentage of subjects reported needing to repeat actions over again. Krupnick (1980) notes impaired concentration in victims of violent crimes who manifest PTSD symptomatology. Similar difficulties have been found in other PTSD patient populations. Residents near Three Mile Island demonstrated significant deficits on task performances (that measure concentration and motivation) when compared to control groups even after one and a half years (Baum, Gatchel & Schaffer, 1983) and almost 5 years (Davidson & Baum, 1986) after the accident.

Irritability/Outbursts of Anger/Rage. Irritability, anger, rage, hostility, and feelings of violence are common features in populations that have endured extreme traumatization.

> Increased irritability may be associated with sporadic and unpredictable explosions of aggressive behavior, even upon minimal or no provocation. The latter symptom has been reported to be particularly common of war veterans with this disorder. (American Psychiatric Association, 1980, p. 237)

As noted above, explosive rage and a tenuous hold on violent impulses have often been noted in Vietnam combat veterans manifesting PTSD (Wilmer 1982c; Lifton, 1982; Goodwin, 1980; Kolb & Mutilipassi, 1982). With respect to Vietnam veterans Walker (1981a) notes that in the early 1980s: 29,000 veterans were incarcerated in state and federal prisons, 37,500 were on parole, 250,000 were on probation, and 87,000 were awaiting trial.

He notes that 70% of all incarcerated veterans had honorable discharges. What is more, incarcerated Vietnam veterans were less likely to have a history of juvenile or adult history of incarceration than their nonveteran counterparts. The conclusion is that the experience of the war contributed significantly towards the development of angry reactions. Rage is commonly experienced in relationship to (Howard, 1975; Walker & Nash, 1981; Shatan, 1973, 1978) (1) authorities; (2) those who have been/are unsupportive; (3) scapegoating; (4) the sense of betrayal; (5) feelings of humiliation; (6) feelings of being deceived; and (7) feelings of being duped and/or manipulated. The problem of rage was compounded in Vietnam veterans by various aspects of the war. These include (Shatan 1978, Goodwin, 1980) (1) encouragement of anger/rage in pre-combat training; (2) military rage part of "masculine identity"; (3) when buddy killed, no enemy to express rage directly toward.

Penk et al. (1981) report significant differences in the ability to control temper between noncombat and combat troops, and between combat troops with varying degrees of combat exposure. What was a "normal" psychological set for the Vietnam war was maladaptive upon return to the U.S. (Shatan, 1978).

Clearly many of these same phenomenon were common for survivors of the holocaust, especially the inability to express rage at the time at which it was felt most strongly. Bychowski (1968) notes that tremendous rage is also commonly found in concentration camp survivors. He notes that the conditions in the death camps promoted "serious characterological derangement" and a "corruption of the superego." Lifton (1967) reports similar feelings among the survivors of the atomic bomb explosions in Japan.

Horowitz et al. (1980) note that anger and hostility are commonly found in patients with stress response syndromes. Feeling easily annoyed and/or irritated was noted in over 80% of subjects. Over 40% of subjects reported:

- temper outbursts that could not be controlled.
- getting into frequent arguments.
- having the urge to break and/or smash things.

Shouting or throwing things and having urges to beat, injure, or harm someone were noted in smaller proportions of the study sample of patients with PTSD.

Krupnick (1980) lists "rage at source of upset" among four common themes found in victims of violent crimes. She argues that the phenomenon of victimization leads to feelings of outrage. Kinzie (1986) reports family violence, anger, or severe irritability in over 25% of the Cambodian refugees with PTSD he studied. Wilkinson (1983) reports anger in about 35% of survivors of the Hyatt Regency Hotel disaster. He notes:

> Natural disasters are viewed as catastrophes totally beyond the individual's or community's control, and the anger that is expressed is often displayed and expressed towards the people who are offering help. However, when the disaster is the result of negligence, apparent indifference, or human failings, the anger is much more intense and focused. (p. 1138)

Wilkinson (1983) notes anger in survivors towards the engineers and designers of the building, the construction workers, and the hotel corporation, as well as toward lawyers, doctors, rescuers, and media personnel.

The feelings of anger, hostility, rage, and violence are not infrequently disturbing to the patient (Krupnick, 1980; Goodwin, 1980). This is especially true when there has been a very real history of violence in the past (e.g., Vietnam combat veterans).

Physiological Reactivity to Events Resembling/Symbolizing Event and the Startle Response. Physiological arousal and the existence of startle responses have been frequently noted with respect to those who have experienced a traumatic event (Kardiner, 1941; Dobbs & Wilson, 1961). The physiological reactivity of patients with PTSD to events evoking the original trauma have been clearly shown in the research of Kolb and Mutilipassi (1982) and Blanchard et al. (1982). Experiments with Vietnam veterans using sodium pentothal and exposure to combat sounds indicated a significant percentage manifested a "conditioned-emotion response." Kolb and Mutilipassi (1982) summarize their findings as follows:

- We posit the existence in the responding group of men of an abnormal potential for arousal of the emotions of fright with all its physiological concomitants when exposed to appropriate stimulation.
- We suggest the existence of an ongoing perceptual motor abnormality with regressive impairment of perceptual discrimination and fixation through emotional conditioning to a primitive startle-arousal pattern.
- The physiologic overreactivity probably is mediated through central adrenergic pathways (p. 985)

Blanchard et al. (1982) report significant differences between combat veterans with PTSD and controls on measures of heart rate, systolic blood pressure, forehead EMG, and skin conductance level when exposed to combat sounds. Heart rate was the most discriminating variable. Behavioral approaches to the treatment of PTSD which have used in physiological assessment procedures confirm increased physiological responsiveness in combat veterans (Fairbank et al., 1981; Keane & Kaloupek, 1982; Fairbank & Keane, 1982; McCafferty & Fairbank, 1985). An exaggerated startle response was also found in over 50% of the Cambodian refugees with PTSD studied by Kinzie (1986).

Hyperalertness/Hypervigilance. Hyperalertness and hypervigilance are also common features of PTSD associated with increased physiological arousal. Bychowski (1968) notes that hypersensitivity is a classical symptom in survivors of concentration camps. Hypertension is also commonly found. These features are also found in all other patient populations manifesting PTSD.

Autonomic arousal symptoms can be best understood in terms of learning theory (see p. 128) and psychobiologic models of PTSD (see p. 160). The theories of classical conditioning and stimulus generalization appear tailor-made to explain the increased arousal (e.g., hypervigilance and exaggerated startle response) as well as the physiological reactivity at exposure to events that symbolize or resemble the trauma, especially in the context of extreme trauma. Alternatively, the psychobiological models (De la Pena, 1984; Van der Kolk et al., 1984; Van der Kolk & Greenberg, 1987) that posit alterations in CNS functioning explain many of the autonomic symptoms as alterations in the patient's physiological functioning (e.g., sleep disturbances, memory, and concentration) and arousal (e.g., hypervigilance, irritability, and outbursts of rage).

An extreme form of hypervigilance is found in the "paranoid adaptation to post-traumatic stress" (Hendin, 1984). Most commonly found in veterans, this response includes:

• eternal vigilance in interactions with others.
• a determination to react violently to any perceived hostility.
• the belief that an argument is a prelude to a fight.
• the feeling that it is best to strike first in a powerful way.

Clearly this form of extreme hypervigilance and associated features overlaps with anger and hostility symptoms, also grouped under the rubric of increased arousal. Hendin (1984) notes

> Paranoid adaptations in general are characterized by a refusal to accept blame or responsibility, so it is not surprising that nearly all veterans with this adaptation tend to deny guilt over their combat experiences. (p. 129)

Some veterans manifest enough paranoia to be given a secondary DSM-III diagnosis of paranoid personality disorder. At root is a deep feeling of vulnerability.

SURVIVOR GUILT AND OTHER FORMS OF GUILT

Guilt, either in the form of survivor guilt or other forms, is a common feature in PTSD. However, although it is part of the DSM-III criteria for PTSD, it is not listed in the DSM-III-R criteria. It is included here with the primary symptoms in keeping with historical observations of survivors and the current DSM-III criteria.

"Survivor guilt" may be expressed in the form, "How is it that I survived while others more worthy than I did not?" (Lifton, 1973). Goodwin (1980) emphasizes that survivor guilt is not a hypothetical construct, but one based on the "harshest of realities." In support of this, Wikler (1981) notes that many booby traps in Vietnam were rigged so that the man who tripped the wire killed not himself but a fellow soldier.

Lifton (1967) notes survivor guilt in hibakusha (survivors of the atomic bombs in Hiroshima and Nagasaki). In addition, survivors often report guilt related to fantasies of having contributed to the cause of the disaster, and responsibility over the deaths of others. Krupnick (1980) notes feelings of responsibility in cases of PTSD among violent crime victims. "This is the belief, however irrational, that one has caused or failed to prevent the event from occurring and is therefore responsible" (p. 348).

Ayalon (1983) found that Israeli children who survived terrorist attacks and were slightly injured experienced less shame and survivor guilt than children who were totally unharmed after the rescue. The explanation was that the slight injuries assuaged the guilt for being "unharmed."

Self-punishment often results from these feelings of responsibility (Krupnick, 1980). Shatan (1978) notes in relation to Vietnam veterans:

> They invite self-punishment by picking self-defeating fights, inviting rejection from near ones, even getting involved in a remarkably high number of single-car, single-occupant accidents. (p. 48)

In support of this, Nefzger (1970) notes that in epidemiological studies of World War II and Korean War POWs high rates of violent death from homicide, suicide, and automobile accidents were indicated.

Generally, the issue of guilt and survivor guilt is discussed in the context of survivors feeling unrealistically guilty. However, there are situations when patients suffering with PTSD in fact have reasons to feel guilty.

As part of their study, Breslau and Davis (1987) evaluated 42 Vietnam veterans who did not participate in wartime atrocities and 27 Vietnam veterans who did participate in atrocities (mostly multiple incidents). All of the men who committed atrocities were diagnosed as having PTSD. The experience of participating in atrocities increased the probability of being given a diagnosis of PTSD by 42% when the number of combat stressors was held constant. The authors suggest that their findings indicate that "reexpereinced" trauma may not necessarily be the most salient experiences of a PTSD patient. These experiences may act like "screen memories" which hide less tolerable experiences.

A related issue to survivor guilt is the phenomenon of self-blame; a common reaction following different times of trauma and victimization, such as rape, battering, disease, and accidents (Janoff-Bulman, 1985). A controversy exists over the functionality of self-blame. Janoff-Bulman (1985) discusses previous research (Bulman & Wortman, 1977) that in paralyzed victims' blame of others was associated with poor coping, and self-blame was a predictor of good coping. Janoff-Bulman (1985) tries to resolve the inconsistency between the view that self-blame can be adaptive and the views that self blame leads to depression (e.g., Beck [[1967]]) by proposing that there are two types of self-blame: behavioral self-blame and characterological self-blame.

Behavioral self-blame is viewed as adaptive. It focuses on specific behaviors the person did or did not do. The important issue with behavioral self-blame is that this type of attribution results in a perceived sense of modifiability and controllability. The traumatic event is attributed to specific behaviors that can be changed through the individual's efforts. Therefore, the trauma can be avoided in the future.

The maladaptive response is termed characterological self-blame. If a person engages in characterological self-blame he or she makes the attribution that the reason something bad happened was due to some enduring character trait which is not modifiable. The characterological self-blamers focus on the past and the question of whether they deserved the trauma or not. Behavioral self-blamers focus on the future and on future avoidability.

Veronen and Kilpatrick (1983) and Kilpatrick (personal communication, March 1988) have found little evidence of characterological self-blame in their extensive work with rape victims. On the other hand, we have had several cases in which characterolical self-blame was clearly evident. It was also fairly clear that the self-blaming was a process that existed before the rape. Finally, our patients who engaged in characterological self-blaming appeared to use the experience of being raped, as *further* evidence of their unworthiness.

At this point, it would be clinically useful to be aware of the two different styles of self-blaming. The hypothesis that can be tentatively offered is that characterological self-blame is just what its name implies, namely, a characterological style of self-accusatory statements. It is not a function of PTSD or victimization per se. However, if someone who tends to engage in characterological self-blaming is victimized, they will have used the same attributional style to cope with the victimization.

The maladaptive style of blaming "the self" will become an important therapeutic issue.

SUMMARY

The primary symptoms of PTSD are those contained in the DSM-III and DSM-III-R criteria. An understanding of the specific symptom clusters required for diagnosis, as well as the many observations in the literature which flesh out these phenomenon, contribute significantly toward the ability to properly assess and positively diagnose PTSD. In the next chapter those clinical phenomenon commonly associated with PTSD, but which are not considered central, are considered.

3

Secondary Symptoms

INTRODUCTION

Usually the clinical picture presented by patients with PTSD is not restricted to those symptoms and clusters outlined in the diagnostic criteria. An understanding of secondary features of the disorder is important for a variety of reasons. First, it promotes a more total understanding of the patient's problems and difficulties, and thus aids in treatment planning and more holistic therapeutic intervention.

Second, since patients may present with secondary features of the disorder, an awareness of those symptoms that may be associated with the disorder enhances assessment procedures and the detection of PTSD where it might otherwise be missed. It is not uncommon for persons presenting with vague dysphoric or depressive features to reveal traumatic events which play a central role in their difficulties.

Third, many of the primary symptoms of PTSD interact with and are influenced by secondary symptom clusters. For example, heightened (general) anxiety significantly impacts upon nearly all of the primary symptom clusters, despite the fact it is not listed in the criteria. Indeed, PTSD often overlaps and/or is coexistent with other DSM-III diagnoses.

Finally, given the very real possibility of future revisions of the Diagnostic and Statistical Manual, symptoms currently regarded as "secondary" may emerge later as "primary symptoms." This has already occurred with respect to "irritability and outbursts of anger" which was not listed in the DSM-III criteria, but is included in the DSM-III-R criteria.

The various secondary features of PTSD have been noted for many years and across all patient populations manifesting PTSD. The most important include depression, anxiety, the presence of a "death imprint" and "death anxiety," impulsive behavior, substance abuse, and somatization. Less commonly noted symptoms include alterations in time sense and various changes in ego functioning.

DEPRESSION/DYSTHYMIC DISORDER

Depression in victims of massive trauma has been a common finding over the years, and is included as an associated feature of PTSD in both the DSM-III and DSM-III-R criteria. Depression has been noted in holocaust survivors (Krystal & Niederland, 1968), survivors of natural disasters (Shore et al., 1986), Cambodian refugees with PTSD (Kinzie, 1986), survivors of the atomic bombings of Hiroshima and Nagasaki (Lifton, 1979), hostages (Sank, 1979), and rape victims (Norris & Feldman-Summers, 1981; Nadelson et al., 1982). Iacono's (1984) factor analysis of PTSD symptoms in Vietnam veterans suggests that depressive features are a major part in the overall factor structure. He recommends that depression be moved from an associated feature to a cardinal feature of the disorder, at least with Vietnam combat veterans. Horowitz et al. (1980) and Wilkinson (1983) note high percentages of depressive features in patients suffering from stress response syndromes. Included in over 75% of those studied were (1) feeling blue; (2) feeling low in energy or slowed down; (3) crying easily; (4) sadness; (5) feeling no interest in things; and (6) feeling hopeless about the future.

Included in over 50% of respondants were (1) feelings of worthlessness; (2) loss of sexual interest or pleasure; (3) fatigue; and (4) recurrent depressive feelings (often frightening). Suicidal thoughts, loss of appetite, and loss of enthusiasm were reported in about 45% of patients.

Despite clinical observations and research support of depression as a frequent symptom of PTSD, it was not included as a cardinal symptom in the diagnostic criteria for PTSD in the DSM-III nor the DSM-III-R. However, many of the cardinal features of PTSD may be regarded as indicative or, or exacerbated by, underlying depression. This includes numbing of responsiveness; reduced involvement, sleep disturbances, and memory impairments/difficulty concentrating.

Frequently the overlapping and simultaneous occurrence of PTSD and depression are found (Shore et al., 1986; Kinzie, 1986). Hence, an awareness of and attendance to depression is a crucial aspect of the assessment and understanding of the broader clinical picture of PTSD. Felt helplessness (Seligman, 1967) is a common finding among traumatized individuals. Of critical importance is the fact that, at least in Vietnam combat veterans with PTSD, the possibility of suicide is always present (Goodwin, 1980). Shatan (1982) notes high rates of suicide among veterans. Krupnick (1980) also notes high suicide rates among victims of violent crimes. With respect to diagnosing patients with PTSD, depressive syndromes should also be indicated.

ANXIETY

As with depression, anxiety has also been noted over the years as a manifestation of post-traumatic symptomatology, and is also included as an associated feature of PTSD in both the DSM-III and DSM-III-R criteria. Again, generalized anxiety, panic disorders, and other anxiety conditions are frequently superimposed on the PTSD. Horowitz et al. (1980) note that the following were reported by over 75% of the patients with stress response syndromes in their study: feeling tense/keyed up, nervousness/shakiness inside, and feeling fearful. Over 50% of patients reported: heart pounding/racing or becoming suddenly scared for no reason.

Anxiety responses have been indicated in all patient populations with PTSD symptoms: hostages (Sank, 1979), natural disasters (Shore et al., 1986), manmade disasters (Smith et al., 1986), etc. Various "anxiety equivalents" were noticed in concentration camp survivors (Krystal & Niederland, 1968). These included (1) heart palpitations; (2) hyperhidrosis (excessive sweating); (3) hyperventilation; and (4) other forms of CNS overactivity. As with depressive syndromes, anxiety conditions should be given a separate diagnosis if they coexist with PTSD symptomatology.

DEATH IMPRINT/DEATH ANXIETY

Lifton (1979; Lifton & Olson, 1976) notes that death imprint and death anxiety are cardinal features of survivors of massive traumatization. The concept of death imprint has relevance for the intrusive imagery found in patients manifesting PTSD. Lifton (1979) defines it specifically as "the radical intrusion of an image-feeling of threat or end to life" (p. 169). Lifton adds,

> [T]he death imprint in traumatic syndrome simultaneously includes actual death anxiety (the fear of dying) and anxiety associated with death equivalents (especially having to do with disintegration of the self). This powerful coming together of these two levels of threat may be the most characteristic feature of image-response in the traumatic syndrome. (p. 170)

Hence, the death imprint encompasses a specific form of intrusion, placing a fundamental emphasis upon death imagery. Indeed, Lifton (1979) speaks of an "indelible image" associated with the death experience. In describing the death imprint in survivors of the Buffalo Creek disaster Lifton and Olson (1976) note: "The memories of destruction were all-encompassing, so that a sense very close to 'it was the end of time' was present in many survivors" (p. 2). Not uncommonly the death imprint produces a "permanent inner terror." Encompassed in the concept is the fear that the trauma will recur. The shattering of a sense of invulnerability is also important.

IMPULSIVE BEHAVIOR

According to the DSM-III, "Impulsive behavior can occur, such as sudden trips, unexplained absences, or changes in life-style or residence" (American Psychiatric Association, 1980, p. 237).

SUBSTANCE ABUSE

Whereas substance abuse was considered possible in the DSM-III description of PTSD, the DSM-III-R description indicates that psychoactive substance use disorders are common complications of the disorder. High incidents of drug abuse have been noted among Vietnam veterans with PTSD (Goodwin, 1980; Wilmer, 1982c).

In an important study of Vietnam veterans that examines the relationship between traumatic neurosis and alcoholism, Lacoursiere et al. (1980) note that many of the symptoms of classical traumatic neurosis can be suppressed through alcohol use. The results appear to be generalizable to other patient populations with PTSD, and other types of substance abuse. Self-medication with alcohol is effective in inducing sleep, reducing anxiety, easing muscle tension, and suppressing REM sleep (with which many post-traumatic nightmares are associated). In some cases it is effective in lifting depression. Initially alcohol use is an effective means of reducing symptoms. However, with continued use tolerance promotes increased consumption. The result is alcoholism superimposed on the original PTSD. With time the use of alcohol becomes less and less effective in reducing the troubling symptoms and may indeed exacerbate them. Lacoursiere et al. (1980) note that the development of alcoholism is secondary to PTSD. Goodwin (1980) notes that substance abuse in veterans is often exaggerated during depressive episodes. Self-medication was a coping response learned in Vietnam.

SOMATIZATION/TENSION

In studies of concentration camp survivors, somatic disorders and psychosomatic disease were found to be frequent (Niederland, 1968; Krystal & Niederland, 1968). Common forms of somatization and tension included:

* excessive tenseness (chronic muscle tension)
* exhaustion/tiredness from the above
* pain in muscle joints
* arthritic-like attacks
* headaches (tension, migraine, "survivor type")
* allergenic symptoms
* peptic ulcers
* gastric overactivity
* colitis
* respiratory syndromes
* cardiac syndromes
* hypochondriasis

Horowitz et al. (1980) also report somatization symptoms in patients suffering from stress response syndromes. Symptoms which occurred in over 75% of subjects included: headaches or feeling weak in various parts of the body. Somatization symptoms occurring in over 50% of patient included:

* nausea/upset stomach
* soreness in muscles
* hot/cold spells
* pains in lower back
* faintness/dizziness
* numbness/tingling in various parts of the body
* heavy feelings in limbs
* lump in throat
* pains in heart/chest

Trouble catching one's breath was noted in over 40% of respondents.

Burgess and Holmstrom (1974) note a number of somatic reactions following rape. These include: skeletal muscle tension, gastrointestinal irritability, and genitourinary disturbance. The severity of somatic reactions varied from patient to patient. These symptoms persisted for several days to several weeks following rape.

ALTERATIONS IN TIME SENSE

The DSM-III-R criteria for PTSD include the sense of a foreshortened future. Terr (1983b) notes a variety of other alterations in time sense following massive psychic trauma. Although these alterations do not occur with the frequency of other PTSD symptoms, their presence may suggest PTSD in cases where the diagnosis was not suspected, or aid in the understanding of the effects of massive trauma on a given patient. In a study involving both children and adults the following time distortions and related post-traumatic phenomena were noted:

- *Misperceptions of time duration:* Patients may report that time seemed to slow down during short traumatic events or speed up during protracted trauma.
- *Gross confusion of sequencing:* Particularly with children, memories of the traumatic event may be confused with reference to time sequence.
- *Time skew:* Events that occurred during the trauma were placed prior to it, with a subsequent sense of prediction.
- *Retrospective presifting/omen formation:* These involve "retrospectively formed warnings" and appear to be more common than many other time-alteration phenomena.
- *Sense of prediction:* The sense that dreams could be predictive, that patients now had psychic abilities.

Terr (1983b) emphasizes that many of the alterations in time sense are attempts on the part of the patient to gain some feeling of control in the face of utter helplessness. She describes this as follows:

> [T]he victim, having experienced, during the traumatic event, a complete loss of control over what occurred, now reestablishes a sense of control by finding an omen or by refusing to plan far into the future, always expecting the worst....[T]he traumatized person now experiences weird sensations of prediction; supernatural purposes; powers of thoughts, wishes, and dreams; burdens of guilt and responsibility; and belief in living only from day to day. (p. 260)

Certainly an understanding of alterations in time sense puts flesh on the bones of the PTSD criteria.

CHANGES IN EGO FUNCTIONING

In his observations of concentration camp survivors, Niederland (1968) notes profound personality changes "showing a more or less radical disruption of the entire maturational development, behavior, and outlook" (p. 13). Lindy and Titchener (1983) note that a number of character changes have been neglected in the formulation of the PTSD criteria. Their orientation is predominantly psychoanalytic and their observations were made with reference to the survivors of the Buffalo Creek Disaster and Vietnam combat veterans. Changes in ego-functioning which result from the development of PTSD include:

- *Overcontrol:* Characteristic defenses are used excessively to ward off intrusive thoughts, feelings, images, and memories.
- *Regression:* Traits not associated with the premorbid character assume a central locus.
- *Rigidity/brittleness of character traits:* Lack of flexibility in use of defensive operations; defenses breakdown under stress.
- *Decrease in repertoire of available resources.*
- *Specific failures in the channeling of hostile impulses:* The ability to sublimate decreases after the trauma.
- *Psychic conservatism:* The patient withdraws from new challenges, avoids "the opportunity for epigenetic maturation of intrapsychic structures."
- *Post-traumatic decline:* This includes a "negative spiraling" between negative changes in character structure, poor management of tension states, and damaged object relations.

Lindy and Titchener (1983) note that the above changes in ego functioning become chronic if immediate intervention is not available to victims.

MISCELLANEOUS SECONDARY FEATURES

Other secondary symptoms of PTSD include adjustment problems, disrupted interpersonal functioning, pronounced sexual difficulties, secondary mental illness, minor/significant alterations in life-style, intense feelings of mistrust, feelings of being betrayed, feelings of being scapegoated, regression, disrupted self-image (activation of "negative self-images").

Each unique traumatic situation also produces its own characteristic associated features. Individuals also develop secondary symptoms depending upon their own character structure and personality makeup.

SUMMARY

The symptoms of PTSD are a function of the person's attempt to cope with events that cannot be experienced, processed and mastered in an adaptive manner using the usual modes of coping. There are multiple theoretical formulations of the nature of PTSD that will be presented in Chapter 6. At this point we will present a summary of the symptoms as described by DSM-III-R. In addition, we will present the most common theoretical orientations that offer a mechanism for the specific symptoms.

4

Subtypes and Course
of the Disorder

In addition to an understanding of the primary and secondary symptoms of PTSD, awareness of the various subtypes and course of the disorder are necessary for assessment and diagnostic procedures.

SUBTYPES

PTSD is not considered a uniform diagnostic category, but one which exibits several subtypes. As delineated in the DSM-III-R these are "PTSD, acute," "PTSD, chronic," and "PTSD, delayed." The latter two subtypes are subsumed under one diagnostic reference number and labeled as "PTSD, chronic or delayed," which includes clinical manifestations of the disorder that could be described as PTSD, delayed and chronic. Table 4.1 illustrates the various subtypes of PTSD possible. Kolb and Mutalipassi (1982) suggest an additional subtype of PTSD which they term "the conditioned emotional response." Each of these is briefly noted.

PTSD, Acute. As noted in the DSM-III:

> Symptoms may begin immediately or soon after the trauma...When symptoms begin within 6 months of the trauma and have not lasted for more than 6 months, the acute subtype is diagnosed and the prognosis is good." (American Psychiatric Association, 1980, p. 237)

Table 4.1. Subtypes of Post-Traumatic Stress Disorder

| | | Onset of symptoms within six months of traumatic event? | |
		Yes	No
Duration of symptoms longer than six months?	No	PTSD, acute	PTSD, delayed
	Yes	PTSD, chronic	PTSD, delayed and chronic

This is the most common form of PTSD. The delayed forms of the disorder are less frequent, although not uncommon as recent literature has established. The prognosis for other subtypes of PTSD is apparently less favorable.

PTSD, Chronic. "PTSD, chronic" is indicated when the duration of symptoms has exceeded 6 months. The choice of 6 months as the demarcation point by the DSM-III and DSM-III-R was essentially arbitrary (Keane, 1988).

Hence, should the symptoms persist for more than 6 months following the traumatic stressing event PTSD, acute must be rediagnosed as PTSD, chronic. PTSD, chronic is subsumed under the label PTSD, chronic or delayed in the DSM-III.

PTSD, Delayed. As noted in the DSM-III, "It is not unusual...for symptoms to emerge after a latency period of months or years following the trauma" (American Psychiatric Association, 1980, p. 237). When symptoms appear 6 months after the stressful event "PTSD, delayed" is indicated. PTSD, delayed is subsumed under the label PTSD, chronic or delayed in the DSM-III.

PTSD, Delayed and Chronic. Although not delineated in the DSM-

III, there is another logical subtype of PTSD: PTSD, delayed and chronic. Such a subtype would refer to clinical presentations in which patients had not develop PTSD symptomatology within the 6 months following the traumatic event (PTSD, delayed), and had manifested PTSD symptoms for a period of greater than 6 months before diagnosis (PTSD, chronic). Many of the PTSD, delayed cases discussed in the literature, might be more accurately described as PTSD, delayed and chronic. For diagnostic purposes the clinical picture of PTSD, delayed and chronic is again subsumed under PTSD, delayed or chronic.

The Conditioned Emotional Response: Subclass of PTSD, Chronic and Delayed. Kolb and Mutalipassi (1982) suggest an additional subtype of PTSD present within the "PTSD, delayed" and "PTSD, chronic" groups. In studies utilizing narcosynthesis (sodium pentathol) the authors delineated a group of combat veterans with PTSD who (1) cognitively dissociated while in a drug altered state of consciousness when exposed to combat sound stimuli, evidencing time regression and acting-out behavior; and (2) developed immediate physiological hyperactivity in both the cardiovascular and neuromuscular systems. They postulate a "conditioned emotional response" which is evident in some patients with PTSD.

Although diagnosis of this subtype of PTSD requires facilities for conducting narcosynthesis and exposing patients to sounds which directly relate to the primary stressor (Kolb & Mutalipassi, 1982), awareness of the strong emotional responses evidenced in some patients—akin to primitive startle responses in infants—can alert clinicians to greater severity of PTSD symptomatology. This subtype of PTSD is not included in the subtypes listed in the DSM-III or DSM-III-R criteria.

COURSE OF THE DISORDER

The course of PTSD has tended to be described with respect to specific subpopulations of patients manifesting the disorder, rather than more generally. In part, this is due to the fact that the various syndromes which are now subsumed under the diagnostic label of PTSD were previously described independently. Certainly there are both similarities and differences in the course of PTSD depending upon the nature and extent of the traumatic event. Here a general outline is provided, followed by various formulations with more specific foci.

An understanding of the course of PTSD is as important as familiarity with the primary symptoms, secondary symptoms, and subtypes of the disorder. Awareness of the temporal characteristics of PTSD aids in assessment, positive diagnosis, treatment planning, and interventions.

General Features

A general outline of the course of PTSD has been provided by Horowitz (1974, 1986). It is not only applicable to most types of PTSD but also explains many of the common symptoms associated with PTSD. Figure 4.2 (derived from the work of Horowitz [1986] and Epstein, [1989]) illustrates this general course of PTSD and related pathological intensifications. The phases of PTSD are:

- *Phase I:* Outcry—The immediate response to the traumatic event (e.g., panic, dissociative reactions, reactive psychoses, stunned uncomprehending daze).
- *Phase II:* Denial—A period of denial and numbing, including maladaptive avoidances (e.g., withdrawal, drug/alcohol abuse, counterphobic frenzy, fugue states).
- *Phase III:* Oscillation between denial/numbing and intrusive thoughts, feelings, images, memories—The intrusive states include flooded and impulsive states, despair, reenactments, etc.
- *Phase IV:* Working through—Intrusions become less intense and more manageable, denial/numbing lifts (anxiety/depressive reaction and physiological disruptions are manifested).
- *Phase V:* Relative completion of response—Likely never reached, the final state includes various permanent alterations in character structure.

Horowitz's (1974, 1986) model of the course of PTSD serves as a cornerstone for the consideration of other conceptualizations. It is general enough to be adapted to the various conditions and time frames under which other phasic reactions to extreme traumatization have been discussed. Two components of the model that need to be differentiated. The first component is the description of the process of the individual attempting to cope with trauma. The essential feature of this process is the alternation between the intrusion of aversive cognitive-affective material and the use of denial and numbing to reduce aversiveness. Clinical and experimental evidence support the idea that this process occurs with the majority of individuals who experience trauma. (The topic will be discussed in more detail in Chapter 5.)

Second, Horowitz's concept of stages (like most other stage theories of reactions to undesirable life events) is more heuristic than empirical.

While we believe that his model can be useful in understanding and treating the symptoms of many individuals with PTSD, it is important that the model not be reified.

In two important reviews of the literature, Silver and Wortman (1980) and Wortman and Silver (1987) have presented strong arguments that challenge many of the assumptions of stage theories in general. A partial summary of their findings includes the following:

1. Most reports that have supported stage theories of reactions to undesirable life events have been merely descriptive, or subjective impressions of interview data or retrospective studies (Silver & Wortman, 1980).
2. Most empirical reports that systematically measure affective states across time produced results that were inconsistent with prevailing stage theories (Silver & Wortman, 1980).
3. The extreme variability of the response patterns to aversive life events does not support the concept of stages of response (Silver & Wortman, 1980).
4. There is an assumption in almost every stage theory that a final stage of resolution exists. However, there is considerable evidence that individuals are not always able to resolve loss in a satisfying manner, particularly if the event is sudden (as in most noncombat PTSD). The time for recovery appears to be much longer than originally expected (Silver & Wortman, 1980; Wortman & Silver, 1987).

While not directly addressing the stage theory of reactions to trauma, Quarantelli (1985) differentiates two styles of evaluating trauma in natural disasters—the individual approach and the social network approach. In doing so, he reports two conflicting sets of findings. The individual approach (Horowitz belongs to this camp) tends to place a great deal of importance on pathological reactions. The social network approach tends to find a great deal of health in populations after a disaster. In the discussion at this point, the implication is that there is not necessarily a single trajectory of phases through which individuals pass after they experience trauma.

Heuristically speaking, it may be more accurate to depict the course of PTSD as having multiple possible trajectories. The branching point appears to occur after Horowitz's phase III. One branch heads in an adaptive fashion, and conforms to Horowitz's model.

Individuals who take this course demonstrate a great deal of adaptability. For some this may reflect the help of psychotherapy, or it may correlate with the responsiveness of the individual and his or her

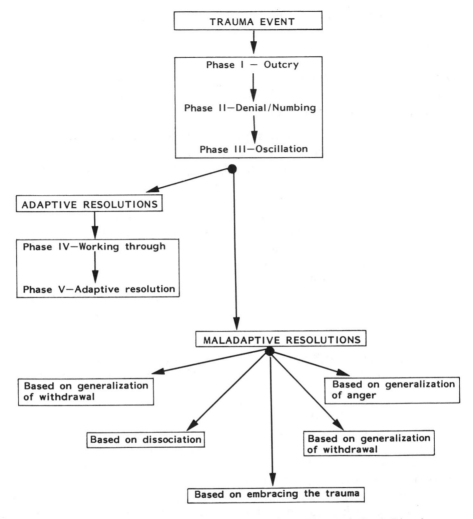

Figure 4.1. Possible Trajectories in the Course of Post-Traumatic Stress Disorder

support system. Epstein (1989) has described the general characteristics of an adaptive resolution. Again, it should be pointed out that these characteristics are descriptive and theoretical.

The second path is a maladaptive resolution of PTSD. According to Epstein (1989), the maladaptive resolution can take one of five forms with the following characteristics:

1. Resolution based on generalization of fear response
2. Resolution based on generalization of the anger response
3. Resolution based on generalization of the withdrawal response
4. Resolution based on dissociation
5. Resolution based on embracing the trauma

The concept of "maladaptive *resolution*" is helpful because it underscores the fact that individuals with chronic PTSD are not simply stuck in an oscillation between denial and intrusions. In an attempt to come to terms with trauma people alter their beliefs about themselves, others, the world, and the best manner to cope with stress (Epstein, 1989). The rigidity of the personality changes, no matter how maladaptive, that are often seen in chronic cases of PTSD can be viewed as evidence that some type of "resolution" has been reached.

Epstein's elaboration has several potential advantages. First, the differentiation of the alternate resolutions can lead to a more accurate diagnosis (beyond simple DSM-III-R classification). Second, the description of the different resolutions suggests that a differentiation of therapeutic interventions is required. Third, with increased specificity of diagnosis, more accurate research can be performed.

Before moving on to describe the courses of PTSD in specific contexts, we suggest that clinicians keep two caveats in mind. First, despite the fact that there is a paucity of "empirical" evidence for Horowitz's description of stages, the depiction does appear to fit many people.

Second, these descriptions are guidelines, rough and incomplete maps of the territory. If they help you understand your patients, use them. If a particular patient does not fit the map, either modify the map or put it away. Clinicians can inadvertently disrupt the therapeutic alli-

---

Table 4.2. Beliefs and Symptoms in Successfully Resolved Trauma[a]

A. Beliefs
  1. World may be unpredictable with some danger and uncontrollablity, *within limits*.
  2. Self is sometimes weak and helpless, *within limits*.
  3. Others are sometimes dangerous, uncaring, weak or untrustworthy, *within limits*.
  4. Ways to cope: varied, flexible, discriminating, and accepting of others; assimilation & accommodation.

B. Symptoms and Positive Consequences
  1. Residual sensitivity to trauma-related cues
  2. Reduced security
  3. Increased awareness. A "sadder but wiser person" who has come to terms with some existential aspects of living, such as vulnerability, suffering, death, good and evil; independence and relatedness.

[a]Adapted from Epstein (1990).

**Table 4.3. Beliefs and Symptoms
in Maladaptive Resolutions of the Traumatic Neurosis[a]**

I. *Resolution Based on Generalization of the Fear Response*
   A. Predominant Beliefs
      1. World is dangerous
      2. Self is weak and vulnerable
      3. Others are dangerous or unhelpful
      4. Ways to cope: vigilance and escape
   B. Symptoms
      1. Hyperalertness to danger of all kinds
      2. Sensitivity to trauma-relevant cues
      3. Chronic anxiety and elevated arousal
      4. Psychosomatic symptoms

II. *Resolution Based on Generalization of the Anger Response (Moving against Others)*
   A. Predominant Beliefs
      1. World is malevolent
      2. Self has been mistreated, exploited, deceived, or betrayed
      3. Others are unjust and untrustworthy
      4. Ways to cope: be strong, defend self, attack enemies
   B. Symptoms
      1. Paranoid suspiciousness
      2. Antisocial acting out

III. *Resolution Based on Generalization of the Withdrawal Response (Moving Away from Others)*
   A. Predominant Beliefs
      1. World is dangerous, ungiving, and uncontrollable
      2. Self is unworthy, unlovable, and self-sufficient
      3. Relationships with others are dangerous
      4. Ways to cope: reject others, rely on own resources
   B. Symptoms
      1. Withdrawal
      2. Alienation
      3. Incapacity for intimacy

IV. *Resolution Based on Dissociation*
   A. Predominant Beliefs (two belief systems)
      1. Dominant belief system: (same as before trauma, but with belief that trauma-relevant cues should be avoided)
      2. Dissociated belief system: (same as for unresolved trauma)
   B. Predominant Symptoms
      1. Dominant system: (normal, except for constriction of behavior and affect)
      2. Dissociated system: (same as for unresolved trauma)

V. *Resolution Based on Embracing the Trauma*
   A. Predominant Beliefs
      1. World is dangerous, malevolent, and lacking in meaning
      2. Self is unloveworthy and lacking in purpose
      3. Others are untrustworthy and objects to be manipulated
      4. Ways to cope: avoid commitment, seek thrills, surmount fear by courting danger, change passive to active
   B. Symptoms
      1. Unreasonable risk-taking
      2. Antiphobic behavior, seeking out trauma-relevant activities
      3. Lack of commitment and direction
      4. Inability to establish intimate relationships

[a]From Epstein (1990). Reprinted by permission.

ance and cause iatrogenic harm when they directly or indirectly communicate that a patient is not going through "the stages" in the "correct manner" (Wortman & Silver, 1987). For example, many patients who have suffered an irrevocable loss are quite capable of expressing positive emotions. It is not a foregone conclusion that they are in the denial or numbing phase (Wortman & Silver, 1987). Clinicians would need to assess the patients' appraisal of their situation. Do they accurately appreciate their situation? Are they capable of changing focus to more dysphoric material when appropriate?

Course of the Disorder in Victims of Military Combat

Frederick (1985) outlines the following phases as characteristic of PTSD in combat veterans:

- *Phase I:* initial impact
- *Phase II:* resistance/denial
- *Phase III:* acceptance/repression
- *Phase IV:* decompensation
- *Phase V:* trauma mastery and recovery

The distinguishing feature of Frederick's (1985) delineation of the course of PTSD in Vietnam combat veterans is the inclusion of a period of decompensation prior to mastery. It may be hypothesized that in situations in which multiple experiences of extreme traumatization are found (i.e., the Vietnam combat arena, death camps, etc.) a period of decompensation may accompany or follow the period of oscillation [Phase III in Horowitz's (1974, 1986) model].

Course of the Disorder in Rape/Assault Victims

Rape is the sine qua non of the type of violent victimization that is likely to lead to the development of PTSD. A well-designed epidemiological study on the development of crime-related PTSD (Kilpatrick et al.,1989) found that among different types of crime (e.g., rape, assault and burglary), completed rape was the only type of crime that predicted the development of PTSD. In fact, 57% of all completed rape victims in the study developed PTSD, and 16.5% still had diagnosable PTSD when assessed an average of 17 years post-rape.

Although PTSD was not recognized as a specific diagnostic category until 1980, Burgess and Holmstrome (1974) developed the concept of the "rape trauma syndrome." They divided the course of rape trauma syndrome into two phases:

- *Phase I:* the acute phase—disorganization
- *Phase II:* the long-term process—reorganization.[3]

Each of these phases has certain characteristics.

The Acute Phase—Disorganization. Phase I of Burgess and Holmstrom's (1974) description of the course of rape trauma syndrome includes three components which appear roughly chronologically: impact reactions, somatic reactions, and emotional reactions.

Impact Reactions. Burgess and Holmstrom (1974) noted that immediately following sexual assault women experience a wide variety of emotions. "The impact of the rape may be so severe that feelings of shock or disbelief are expressed" (p. 982). However, they suggested that there are two basic response styles. The first pattern they term the "expressive style." Women who react according to this pattern typically express their fear, anger, and anxiety through crying, sobbing, smiling, restlessness, and tenseness. The second pattern is termed the "controlled style." Women for whom this style is characteristic tend to mask their feelings, appear calm and composed, and to subdue their affective response. Burgess and Holmstrom (1974) note that, based on their research sample, women tend to present these two basic styles in approximately equal numbers.

Somatic Reactions. Burgess and Holmstrom (1974) note that in the weeks following sexual assault women evidenced many somatic reactions. They noted the following as particularly evident:

- *Physical trauma:* This includes soreness and bruising which resulted directly from the attack; for women forced to have oral sex with their assailants throat irritation and trauma were noted
- *Skeletal muscle tension:* Manifestations of chronic skeletal muscle tension including tension headaches, startle reactions, fatigue, and sleep disturbances
- *Gastrointestinal irritability:* Nausea, stomach pains, and loss of appetite were common symptoms
- *Genitourinary disturbance:* Following rape common gynecological symptoms include vaginal discharge, itching, a burning sensation on urination, and generalized pain as well as chronic vaginal infections and rectal pain and bleeding in victims forced to have anal sex

Kilpatrick, Veronen & Best (1985) reported that in their sample of rape victims common physiological reactions included shaking or trembling, heart racing, pain, tight muscles, and rapid breathing.

Emotional Reactions. The emotional reactions to rape are manifold. The emotional descriptions used by the vast majority of women include feeling scared, worried, terrified, and helpless (Kilpatrick, Veronen & Best, 1985). Perhaps the most commonly experienced emotion is fear, especially since many rape victims report that they were especially fearful of physical violence and death during the assault. Humiliation, embarrassment, anger, guilt, shame, and revenge are also common. Because our culture still too often conceptualizes rape as "being the woman's fault," feelings of self-blame are often induced or amplified.

The Long-Term Process—Reorganization. Burgess and Holmstrom (1974) note the development of the following types of fears:

- *Fear of indoors:* This phobia is particularly common in women who were attacked while sleeping in their own beds.
- *Fear of outdoors:* Women who were attacked outside of their homes are prone to develop a phobia of the outdoors; not infrequently these women feel safer indoors and when traveling outside the home while in the presence of another person.
- *Fear of being alone:* Almost all of the victims report fears of being alone following sexual assault.
- *Fear of crowds:* Phobic reactions to crowds appear to reflect a discomfort with people's physical contact.
- *Fear of people behind them:* When a woman had been approached from behind by her assailant the phobic fear of people behind her is more likely to develop.
- *Sexual fears:* A very common reaction to rape is the severe disruption of the normal sexual pattern of victims; this is particularly difficult for women who were not sexually active before the attack.

The common and more idiosyncratic fears of rape victims appear to follow the laws of classical conditioning, as long as one recognizes that cognitive events can also become conditioned stimuli or cues that elicit anxiety (Veronen & Kilpatrick, 1983).

Burgess and Holmstrom (1974) note that the second phase in the course of rape trauma syndrome is marked by attempts at reorganization. This characterization complements the view of attribution theory and the importance of cognitive appraisal in the recovery process from rape. The essential adaptive task for rape victims is to attribute meaning to the experience in such a manner that their lives are reorganized in a positive direction (Veronen & Kilpatrick, 1983).

One might ask, "How long is the "acute phase" of the syndrome?" Burgess & Holmstrom (1974) suggested that while there were individual differences, the typical length of time was 2 to 3 weeks. Interpreting the data from Kilpatrick, Veronen and Best (1985), and Veronen and Kilpatrick (1983), one potential answer is between 1 week to 1 month. Up to 1 month after the rape, victims were significantly more disturbed than nonvictims on 25 of 28 measures. At 3 months post-rape, the level of distress had subsided significantly; victims only scored significantly higher than nonvictims on measures of fear and anxiety (Veronen & Kilpatrick, 1983).

The next question one might ask is how long is the long-term phase? The answer here is not so clear. As early as 6–21 days post rape, approximately 25% of victims are coping reasonably well without treatment (Kilpatrick, Veronen & Best, 1985). A significant number of women demonstrate a substantial improvement by 3 months post-rape without treatment (Veronen & Kilpatrick, 1983; Kilpatrick, Veronen & Best, 1985). However, a sizeable proportion of rape victims (16.5%) have PTSD many years after the rape (Kilpatrick et al., 1988).

The data from the longitudinal study of rape victims (Kilpatrick, Veronen & Best, 1985) raises the issue of whether or not it is particularly accurate to think of "*one* rape-trauma syndrome" with two phases. The degree of distress measured at 3 months post-rape remained stable at 4-year follow-up; furthermore, victims distress levels at 6–21 days was highly predictive of distress at the 3-month interval. There were also 4 different groups of victims ranging from low distress to high distress. If in the first 21 days post rape a woman was in high distress, she was likely to be in high distress 4 years later. If a woman was in low distress initially, she was likely to be coping well 4 years later. The implication of these findings supports our contention that there are different trajectories of response to trauma. (See page 000)

At this point it would be reasonable to ask whether or not there are any variables that account for the different types of response to rape. The answer is yes. The most important variable in determining the probability of the development of PTSD is the victim's *cognitive appraisal of being in serious physical danger or loss of life* (Kilpatrick, 1988). The chance of a rape victim developing PTSD increased 2.75 times if she experienced physical injury or life threat. Furthermore, when compared to victims of other crimes who did not experience physical injury or life threat, the rape victim who did experience physical injury or life threat was 8 times more likely to develop PTSD (Kilpatrick et al., 1989).

A second important variable appears to be whether or not the woman is involved in a loving relationship with a man in the year prior to the rape. High distress rape victims were three times more likely not to have had any intimate loving relationship with a man than low distress victims (Kilpatrick, Veronen & Best, 1985). A third variable is the response of "the system" to the rape victim. In one study, *two-thirds of variance* of SCL-90 can be accounted for by the answer to the question assessing satisfaction to the criminal justice system; of course the correlation was negative. The less satisfaction the more the symptoms (Kilpatrick, 1988).

Course of the Disorder in Victims of Accidental Manmade Disasters

Rangell (1976) provides an understanding of the course of psychic trauma following a major disaster. Rangell (1976) notes three phases in the reaction of victims of the Buffalo Creek disaster:

- *Phase I:* psychic numbness
- *Phase II:* "ground" and "surround"
- *Phase III:* future effects of the trauma

Psychic Numbness. Rangell (1976) notes that the first reaction of the inhabitants of Buffalo Creek to the dam break included the flooding of the ego, the "traumatic state," and the condition of psychic helplessness. He describes this as the phase of psychic numbness. Characteristic of this phase are apathy, sluggishness, and withdrawal.

"Ground" and "Surround." Rangell (1976) notes that when an individual confronts a significant stress or loss, he or she generally returns to familiar surroundings. Rangell (1976) refers to these surroundings as the person's "ground," the background of his or her life that provides security and the necessary "nurturing supplies" for the process of integrating the stressful event. However, in the case of the Buffalo Creek disaster and, by extension, other disasters of s similarly devastating nature, the familiar surroundings are destroyed or altered. Consequently, victims must not only face the task of processing the original trauma, but also the challenges of continuing their lives in strange surroundings. The major point Rangell (1976) makes is that "the change from the familiar to a strange surround during the period when rest and nurture were needed superseded the initial trauma and prolonged and compounded its effects in each survivor" (p. 315). This second phase in the course of psychic trauma following a major disaster constitutes a second, quite separate set of traumatic events. Hence, the individual continues to react to overwhelming stress.

Future Effects of the Trauma. Making the point that massive psychic trauma occupies much of the "psychic space" of individuals, Rangell (1976) speculates on the long-term effects of disasters on the mental functioning of survivors. He suggests that at the very least the recurrent thoughts of the disaster will seriously restrict victims' psychic life. Given that survivors of the Buffalo Creek disaster were the victims of a catastrophe which could have been avoided, Rangell (1976) adds that, in comparison to "natural disasters," the human element stimulates impulses of retaliation and aggression. Hence, over time, "The ego is bombarded from two directions, and feelings of rage, impotence, anxiety, guilt, and depression are added to the usual responses to disaster" (p. 315). Rangell (1976) also speculates that traumatic neuroses and psychoneuroses exist in a reciprocal relationship to one another. Thus, immediately following the stressing event, traumatic neuroses dominate the psychological picture. However, as time progresses, the two types of "neurosis" begin to occupy similar amounts of psychic energy, with the traumatic neuroses eventually taking second place to the preexisting psychoneuroses. But what is of further concern is the interactive effect of the traumatic response with the preexisting psychoneuroses.

There exists a second view of the reactions of individuals to disasters. The work of the Disaster Research Center (DRC) as reported by Quarantelli (1985) makes a powerful case for the position that personal and social disorganization necessarily occurring after disasters is not supported by field research. He makes the following points:

1. A differentiation between the demands of the disaster itself (agent demands), such as search and rescue and care for the sick; and the demands created by the activities that follow a disaster (response generated demands), such as communication, ongoing assessment, and maintaining order.

2. The distinction between the individual trauma approach and the social sponge approach. The individual trauma approach holds that because disasters are highly stressful they are traumatic life events that produce pervasive and deeply internalized negative effects on the survivors.

   The social sponge approach holds that community disasters have both positive and negative effects; and, many of the latter are short-lived in duration.

   Communities respond remarkably well to disasters, with little increase in mental illness. Much of the trauma that does occur is a function of what happens *after* the disaster (response generated demands).

3. Five possible reasons are given for discrepancies between the two approaches:

a. Since there has been very little overlap in the specific disasters studied, the researchers may be observing actual differences. This is not viewed as a likely explanation.

b. Differences in data-gathering lead to different inclusion criteria for appropriate data. The social sponge approach tends to use methods appropriate for population surveys. The individual trauma approach tends to use self-selected samples. For instance, the Buffalo Creek data consist of material taken from individuals pressing a lawsuit.

c. Practitioners using the individual trauma approach tend to be clinicians whose objectives are to provide treatment. The social sponge approach is used by researchers looking at the entire social response. The clinicians are interested in the people with "the illness" (in this case, PTSD). But the incidence of the disorder is relatively insignificant from the stand point of statistical research purposes.

d. Researchers can interpret data differently. For instance, in one sample, the Disaster Research Center group found significant evidence of a decrement of "psychological well-being" after the Xenia tornado. However, the Disaster Research Center group reached the conclusion that the tornado had "little significant negative impact on the mental health of the affected population" (p. 199), because they placed emphasis on the finding that on almost all of the behavioral measures, the post-impact figures were the same or lower than comparable pre-impact figures.

e. In many instances there is little differentiation between the type of disasters. It is particularly important to differentiate individual from community disasters and natural from technological disasters.

f. Some of the contradictions between the two schools stem from the fact that they are using different models. The individual trauma approach views disaster from a medical model and the social sponge approach views disaster as a social problem.

It is interesting to note that there is little discussion in the PTSD literature that reflects the arguments raised by Quarantelli (1985). Nevertheless, the finding that communities as a whole do remarkably well in disasters has been noted in the London bombings during World War Two and Hiroshima (Rachman, 1978).

So, what are we as clinicians supposed to make of these conflictual findings? Several conclusions can be reached.

1. While social factors and contextual factors are important variables, PTSD is essentially a "unit" problem.
2. In understanding the etiology of a given person's PTSD, one can place too much emphasis on the stressor. It is more relevant to evaluate the stressor-resource balance. (see p. 000)

Course of the Disorder in Hiroshima Survivors

Although PTSD has been noted in many patient populations, the largest potential population of persons manifesting PTSD symptomatology are those who would be directly or indirectly affected by a nuclear war. Without a doubt large numbers of people would develop PTSD. Lifton (1967) has described the course of PTSD with respect to the hibakusha, the survivors of the atomic bomb dropping on Hiroshima, Japan during World War II. An awareness of the course of PTSD in this set of circumstances is important insofar as mental health professionals may be forced to deal with survivors of nuclear incidents. Lifton (1967) delineates four phases:

- *Phase I:* the overwhelming immersion in death
- *Phase II:* "invisible contamination"
- *Phase III:* later radiation effects ("A-bomb disease")
- *Phase IV:* identification with the dead

The overwhelming immersion in death. As noted earlier with reference to the "death imprint" and death anxiety" (see Chapter 3), Lifton's (1967) focus is on the experience of death. with respect to the bombing of Hiroshima Lifton (1968) notes, "the most significant psychological feature...was the sense of a sudden and absolute change from normal existence to an overwhelming encounter with death" (p. 172). Helplessness and a fear of annihilation were dominant during this first phase. Within seconds or minutes many survivors manifested "psychic closing off"—they ceased to feel.

"Invisible Contamination." In essence, this was the sudden, unexpected manifestation of the symptoms of acute radiation which emerged in a "mysterious way." Included were nausea, vomiting, lesions, etc. Rumors that everyone would be dead within three years, that no vegetation would ever grow in Hiroshima again, and that the city would be uninhabitable for 70 to 75 years contributed to death imagery. Powerful affective responses included:

- fear of epidemic contamination leading to body deterioration

- a profound sense of individual powerlessness
- the sense that the contamination had a supernatural origin

Later Radiation Effects. An exploding nuclear device produces "...a taint of death which attaches itself not only to one's entire psychobiological organism, but to one's posterity as well" (Lifton, 1968, p. 178). The emergence of leukemia, psychosomatic problems, and genetic disorders prolonged the encounter with death for survivors. The most predominant fear was of contaminating future generations.

Identification with the Dead. The final phase in Lifton's (1968) description of hibakusha involves a life-long identification with death, dying, and those who died during the bombing and immediately afterwards. Central to the process of identification is survivor guilt, with powerful feelings that survival was earned because others had died. "The survivors feel compelled to merge with the dead, and, in various ways, to behave as if they too were dead" (p. 179).

The most striking feature of Lifton's (1967) description of the course of PTSD in hibakusha is the fact that there is no "recovery." Like the survivors of the holocaust, the nature and extent of the traumatic event were so profound and beyond conceptualization that a return to previous levels of functioning would be impossible.

Course of the Disorder with Residents of Three Mile Island

Baum, Gatchel and Schaeffer (1983) reported that 17 months after the TMI accident, residents living near the plant evidenced more emotional stress than those living near an undamaged nuclear plant, a coal-fired plant and no plant. They also had more difficulty on task performance. There were also significant elevations of urinary catecholamines, which is a sign of chronic sympathetic arousal. At a 5-year follow-up, Davison & Baum (1986) found that TMI residents still had significant deficits on measures of task performance. There was also evidence of increased systolic and diastolic blood pressure, and heart rate when compared to controls. (However, unlike the earlier study these controls did not live near a power plant.) These measures were included to show signs of chronic stress. On a measure of Post traumatic stress, The Impact of Events Scale (Horowitz, 1986), the TMI residents evidenced more intrusive thoughts and avoidance behaviors than controls.

SUMMARY

An awareness of the general course of PTSD is essential. It provides a central reference point about which descriptions of the course of PTSD in specific subpopulations manifesting the disorder can be understood. Given that each traumatic stressor produces variations on the basic theme, an understanding of the course of PTSD as it relates to specific groups is also required for purposes of assessment, diagnosis, treatment planning, and therapeutic intervention. To this effect various delineations of the course of PTSD in Vietnam veterans, rape victims, and man-made disaster victims were described.

5

PTSD in Children

OCCURRENCE

There has been a growing literature on the subject of PTSD in children. The literature consistently points to children's vulnerability to the development of PTSD after severe trauma. In earlier work, such as the evaluation of the children who survived the Buffalo Creek disaster (Newman, 1976), PTSD per se is rarely discussed. Nevertheless, Newman (1976) reported that most of the 224 children were "significantly or severely emotionally impaired." Examples of symptoms often conformed to one or several diagnostic criteria consistent with PTSD.

The literature after 1980 makes specific reference to PTSD, as well as the high incidence of the disorder. Frederick (1985) evaluated 150 children (50 victims of disasters, 50 victims of physical abuse, and 50 victims of child molestation) for PTSD, using the Reaction Index[4] (see Chapter 7, p. 115 for description). Across all the cases, 77% of the children were diagnosed as having PTSD. In addition, Frederick (1985) states that among 300 cases of child molestation, if the child was above the age of 6 PTSD was *always* in evidence.

The same instrument was used to evaluate 300 adult victims of various trauma (e.g. hostages, human induced catastrophes, and natural disasters). Of the adults, (only) 57% developed PTSD compared to 77% incidence with the children.

Arryo and Eth (1985) found that one-third of 30 children traumatized by warfare in Central America were diagnosed with PTSD according to DSM-III criteria. Kinzie et al. (1986) discovered that 50%

61

of 40 Cambodian children refugees had PTSD four years after leaving Cambodia. Malmquist (1986) reported that 100% of 16 children who witnessed either parental homicide or attempted familicide met DSM-III criteria for PTSD. If violence accompanies the trauma, children are more prone to severe psychological reaction (Frederick, 1985).

SYMPTOMS

Elaborating on her work with 50 traumatized children, including the 25 children of Chowchilla, Terr (1979, 1983, 1985) states that there are six significant differences between PTSD in adult and PTSD in children. These are:

1. Children over the ages of 3 or 4 do not become partly or fully amnesic. They do not employ the denial of reality. They do not employ massive repression.[5]
2. Children, as opposed to adults, do not exhibit psychic numbing.
3. "Children do not experience sudden, unexpected visual flashbacks that interrupt their behavior or concentration...Children do consciously choose to think about their ordeals"...they do not experience what Horowitz(1976) conceives of as alternating pattern of intrusion and massive denial. (p. 52)
4. Children's school performance generally suffers only a few months after the trauma, in contrast to the long-term work problems of many adults.
5. Post-traumatic play and reenactment of the trauma happen much more frequently with children.
6. "Time skew is more common and more dramatically expressed in children." (p. 53)
7. Children often demonstrate a striking foreshortening of their view of the future.

While there is considerable accord with these findings, some authors do not agree with Terr's conclusion that children do not have intrusive imagery. Malmquist (1985) studied 16 children who had witnessed a parental murder or an attempted familicide.[6] He found that the children did have intrusive thoughts. While he did not state that they were visual flashbacks, in response to the Impact of Events Scale (Horowitz, 1986), 88% of the children stated that images popped into their mind. He did find that psychic numbing was not present. In fact, the children tended to be hyperalert and agitated. On the other hand, the children actively avoided thinking or talking about the trauma.

Kinzie et al. (1986) reported on the effects of massive trauma on 40 Cambodian refugee children. Half the children were diagnosed with PTSD. Waking intrusive imagery was not reported in the sample. A marked tendency to deny distress and avoidance of memories or talking about experience was noted.

Nir (1985) describes the prevalence of PTSD in children with cancer. Intrusive recollections and repetitious dreams and nightmares are common reactions in pediatric oncology. He cites Koocher and O'Malley (1981) stating that particular problem with childhood cancer has been termed the Damocles syndrome. The syndrome "describes the omnipresent fear of relapse that haunts the child—no matter how many years have passed since the treatment that produced the cure" (p. 127). The child or the family are particularly vulnerable to react to anything that resembles the disease or to illness in general. The problem of stress reactions has become more apparent as longevity and survival rates of childhood cancer improve.

Frederick (1985) listed the following common signs to alert parents and clinicians to the possibilities of PTSD after periods of crisis:

1. Sleep disturbances that continue for more than several days, wherein actual dreams of the trauma may or may not appear.
2. Separation anxiety or clinging behavior, such as a reluctance to return to school.
3. Phobias about distressing stimuli (e.g., a school building, TV scene or person) that remind the victim of the traumatic event.
4. Conduct disturbances, including problems that occur at home or at school, which serve as responses to anxiety or frustration.
5. Doubts about the self, including comments about body confusion, self-worth, and desire for withdrawal.

All of these findings are reported by other authors: sleep disturbances (Aaryo & Eth, 1985; Kinzie et al. 1986; Malmquist, 1986; Newman, 1976; Nir, 1985), conduct disturbances (Burke et al., 1982; Malmquist, 1986), especially in adolescence (Newman, 1976), separation anxiety (Newman, 1976) phobias to stimuli similar to the trauma (Kinzie et al., 1986; Malmquist, 1986; Newman, 1976), doubts about self-worth (Kinzie et al., 1986).

Finally, Terr (1983, 1985) has described the propensity for traumatized children to see ghosts of family members or friends who died as a result of the traumatic event. She reports that they "see" or "feel" the loved one. She reported that ghosts were only experienced in cases where a traumatic death occurred.

PARENTAL RESPONSES

The response of the parents appears to be an important mediating variable in the child's ability to cope with trauma. In World War II, children were better able to cope when they were able to stay with calm and supportive parents (Freud & Burlingham, 1943). In their work with Cambodian refugees, Kinzie et al. (1986) reported that there was a significant correlation between psychiatric diagnosis (of PTSD or major depression) and current family profile. Thirteen of 14 Cambodian refugee children who did not live with a member of the nuclear family had a psychiatric diagnosis; whereas only 14 of 26 children who lived with at least one member (mother, father or siblings) of the nuclear had a psychiatric diagnosis.

Nir (1985) points out that parental coping response can also become a significant source of stress for children with cancer. One stressful parental style was labeled "aggressive pursuers." These are parents that shop for the "best" treatment often in total disregard of the needs and wishes of the child. "The aggressive pursuer intensifies the traumatic experience of the child as their frenetic activity heightens the child's feelings of vulnerability and undermines his/her trust in the medical establishment" (p. 126).

Parents who employ strong intellectual, obsessive-compulsive mechanisms can intensify the stress of childhood cancer. They tend to become highly involved in the medical situation. They repeatedly check on the oncologist's decisions. Their behavior sets up a defensive and hostile atmosphere with the medical staff. Their behavior also sends a message to the child that the doctors cannot be trusted, which can increase the child's anxiety (Nir, 1985).

Another coping style that can cause additional stress for children with cancer can be seen with certain fathers of adolescent boys with cancer. They behave in macho fashion as an attempt to neutralize their own anxiety.

Conversely, Nir (1985) states that adaptive parental coping response can reduce stress for the child. It was found that parents who could develop a therapeutic alliance with the pediatric oncologist, as well as parents with strong religious beliefs, were best able to buffer the child from the pain and stress of the disease and its treatment.

Parental Underreporting

One pattern that begins to become apparent in the different reports of children's reactions to stress is that the parents do not perceive the children to be in as much pain as the children perceive. Terr (1983) reports that none of the Chowchilla parents sought any counseling for their children and that they consistently downplayed the significance of the kidnapping.

In evaluating the response of 81 preschoolers to a blizzard and flood, Burke et al. (1982) found that while parents scored their children as having negative behavior changes on specific items of a standard school questionnaire, not a single parent indicated that their child's behavior had worsened when asked a global question about their child's reaction to the storm. This was interpreted as parental denial of the impact of the disaster.

Parents of Cambodian survivors of trauma also misperceived the difficulty that their children were having (Sack et al., 1986). However, instead of the explanatory principle of denial, the authors felt the finding was due to the cultural value of bearing pain silently. Children who lived near TMI also reported stronger and more symptomatic responses for themselves than did their parents. Furthermore, when there were personality changes noted, none of the parents attributed this to TMI, whereas half of the children did (Handford et al., 1986).

It is difficult to know the meaning of the tendency for parents not to recognize the difficulties their children are having. While it may be a question of denial, one needs to ask if this denial is significantly different in quantity and quality from parental responses to psychological problems in general. It is also probable that part of the problem is that the children simply do not tell their parents how badly they are feeling. The tendency towards suppression and avoidance has already been noted. It may also be that parents work under the premises of "let sleeping dogs lie, or if it don't squeak don't fix it." Once again, the question arises whether parents of children with different types of problems (e.g., reactions to divorce) are any more accurate in appraising the degree of stress their children are experiencing. In any event the implication of these findings is that data from both the parents and the children are important. Furthermore, when asking parents for evaluations of their children, more specific questions would be better than global assessments.

SUMMARY

While the vast majority of writing on PTSD has been about soldiers, it may be that children are the foremost victims of PTSD. Depending on the type of trauma, incident rates range from 40–100%. Children present many of the same types of symptoms as adults (e.g., sleep disorders, avoidance of activities that resemble the trauma, avoidance of talking or thinking about the trauma), but differ in important manners (e.g., hyperactivity instead of numbing, seeing ghosts, alterations of time sense). Parental response to trauma and to the child's reactions to trauma are important variables in the amelioration or exacerbation of the stress the child experiences.

II

Theories

6

Theoretical Perspectives

INTRODUCTION

A variety of conceptual models have been developed to explain the formation and resultant symptomatic picture of PTSD. Within the field of trauma research the information-processing model advocated by Horowitz (1973, 1974, 1976, 1979), the psychosocial framework outlined by Green, Wilson, and Lindy (1985), and the behavioral/learning theory model suggested by Keane et al. (1985) have been the most influential. Various psychodynamic models put forward ("classical," Eriksonian, and object relations theory) have contributed toward a greater understanding of PTSD as it pertains to the individual and his/her internal functioning. Current psychophysiologic and psychobiologic models of PTSD are also the subject of much interest. Shultz's (1984) cybernetic model of PTSD brings a systems understanding to the disorder.

Each of the aforementioned theoretical positions is briefly described below. Although there is some overlap among the different models, each is delineated individually since the various therapeutic strategies for treating PTSD generally relate to specific models.

AN INFORMATION-PROCESSING MODEL

Perhaps the most influential model for PTSD is the information-processing model proposed by Horowitz (1973, 1974, 1976, 1979, 1986). Keane (personal communication, January 15, 1987) notes that

Horowitz's model has had a major impact in the area of theory. Indeed, this model formed the cornerstone for the diagnostic criteria included in the DSM-III for PTSD.

Horowitz's (1973, 1974) model of PTSD builds upon classical and contemporary theories of trauma, but places a major emphasis on information processing and cognitive theories of emotion. Basic elements of the information processing model include:

- "information" (i.e., ideas, images, affects, etc.)
- a "completion tendency" in which important information is processed until reality and cognitive models match (i.e., the situation must terminate, or the cognitive model must be altered to incorporate the new information)
- "information overload": a situation in which new information cannot be processed
- "incomplete information processing": a state in which new information has only been partially processed and where the information remains in an "active form of memory" out of conscious awareness with concomitant influences on ego functioning

Horowitz (1979) contends that catastrophic events involve massive amounts of internal and external information, most of which cannot be matched with a person's cognitive schemata due to the fact it lies outside the realm of normal experience. The result is information overload; the person experiences ideas, affects, and images which cannot be integrated with the self.

Since a person experiencing extreme traumatization cannot process the information, it is shunted out of awareness. It therefore remains in an unprocessed, active, or raw, form. Denial and numbing are employed as defensive maneuvers to keep the traumatic information unconscious. However, due to the completion tendency (similar to psychoanalytic formulations of the so-called "repetition compulsion") the traumatic information does become conscious at times as part of the process of information processing. "They will produce thought representations of the traumatic event on all levels of cognitive functioning, which sometimes break through as emotionally upsetting, intrusive, and uncontrollable images of the event" (Green, Wilson, & Lindy, 1985, p. 55). "Intrusions" also include flashbacks, repetitive nightmares, unwanted thoughts, and the like. Theoretically such intrusive psychic material continues to enter consciousness until the traumatic information is fully processed. When the ego experiences information overload during intrusive episodes, denial-numbing again comes into play. Hence, there is an oscillation between intrusion and denial-numbing prior to full integration of the traumatic material. This is a naturally occurring feature of information processing (Horowitz & Wilner, 1976).

The focus is therefore on completing the processing of information rather than abreaction and catharsis. Horowitz's (1974) functional perspective regards intrusions as potentially facilitating information processing, and defensive operations as promoting the gradual assimilation of traumatic experience.

> Excessive controls interrupt the process, change the state of the person to some form of denial and may prevent complete processing of the event. Failures to control lead to excessive levels of emotion, flooding, and retraumatization, causing entry into intrusive states. Optimal controls slow down recognition processes and so provide tolerable doses of new information and emotional responses. (Horowitz, 1979, p. 249)

Completion of information processing continues until the new information becomes part of "long-term models and inner schemata" (Horowitz, 1979). Thus, "At completion, the experience is integrated so it is part of the individual's view of the world and of him- or herself, and no longer needs to be walled off from the rest of his or her personality" (Green, Wilson, & Lindy, 1985, p. 56). At this point the trauma is no longer stored in an active state.

Following the above, Horowitz (1974, 1979, 1986) outlines progressive stages in the reaction to massive stress:

- *Phase I:* massive stress→crying out/stunned reaction
- *Phase II:* avoidance (denial and numbing)
- *Phase III:* oscillation period (denial-numbing↔intrusions)
- *Phase IV:* transition
- *Phase V:* integration ("completing the processing of information")

In order to understand the particular symptomatic presentation of a patient, Horowitz (1986) places considerable emphasis on the characterological cognitive style, patterns of conflict, and coping mechanisms of the individual. Furthermore, these factors will influence the choice and style of the therapist's interventions.

For example, patients with hysterical styles will tend to process information in an impressionistic fashion. One reason that completion will not occur is that feelings are given more weight than ideas. In therapy, one of the methods for completing the information processing will be to help the patient think through the ideas systematically. In other words, the people with hysterical styles will need to see more of the trees and less of the forest, if they are to find closure on a stressful event. In contrast, people with obsessional styles will tend to prevent the completion of information processing by jumping between isolated ideas or feelings without seeing the connection. These individuals will need to learn to see more of the forest and less of the trees. Therapists can help these patients by holding them to a particular theme or context (Horowitz 1986).

The information processing model of PTSD (Horowitz, 1974, 1979) is an extension of psychoanalytic concepts of trauma. A catastrophic event continues to influence the psychic equilibrium of a victim until the information generated from that event can be matched to a current cognitive model, or a new model can be generated which can integrate the new information. Hence, symptoms persist until the information is fully processed. Within the context of individual psychodynamic therapy, the model is unsurpassed. Horowitz (1986) demonstrates an impressive ability to modernize analytic concepts.

A PSYCHOSOCIAL FRAMEWORK

The psychosocial model proposed by Green, Wilson, and Lindy (1985) is widely known and accepted in the field of PTSD (see Figure 6.1). Its utilization comes from its focus on the interaction of the traumatic stressor, "normal" reactions to catastrophe, individual characteristics, and the social/cultural environment in which the trauma is experienced and in which the patient recovers. It builds on the information-processing model of PTSD suggested by Horowitz (1976, 1979). At heart this model seeks to account for the fact that certain persons exposed to massive trauma develop PTSD, while others do not.

As Wilson and Krauss (1985) note, a person experiences "psychic overload" until the trauma can be successfully integrated. Psychic overload is defined as "...a state in which the nature, intensity, and meaning of the experience(s) are not readily understandable in terms of existing conceptual schemata of reality" (p. 107). It is the failure of the ego defenses and coping mechanisms in the face of catastrophe which leads to the inability to process the experience. Should the person be in a favorable recovery environment, the possibilities of working through the trauma are enhanced. Similarly, should the environment be unsupportive, the possibility of working through the trauma is reduced.

The Traumatic Experience

Wilson (1983) and Green, Wilson, and Lindy (1985) note that the specific characteristics of the traumatic experience are important in relation to long-term response. Crucial elements include:

- severity of stressor
- duration of trauma
- warning speed of onset
- degree of bereavement
- degree of displacement of person/community
- proportion of the community affected degree of life threat
- exposure to death
- dying destruction combat stress (in veterans)
- participation (including the role taken by the survivor, i.e., passive or active)
- degree of moral conflict potential for and/or control over reoccurrence

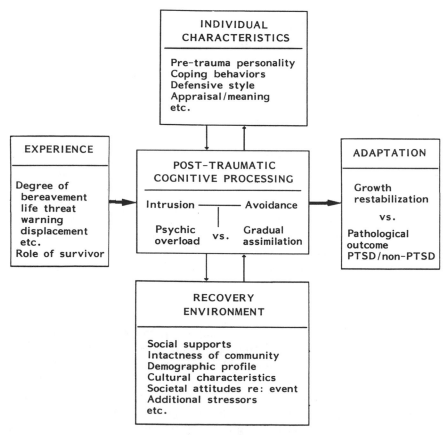

Figure 6.1. Psychosocial Framework for Understanding Post-Traumatic Stress Disorder

The greater frequency of the above leads to a greater likelihood of a survivor developing PTSD. As Wilson and Krauss (1985) argue, the nature of the trauma determines how much information processing will be needed.

Individual Characteristics

Within this interactional model the characteristics of the individual are also important (Wilson, 1977, 1978; Green, Wilson & Lindy, 1985). Variables considered as salient include (1) ego-strength; (2) effectiveness/nature of coping resources/defenses; (3) presence of preexisting psychopathology; (4) prior stressful/traumatic experiences; (5) behavioral tendencies; and (6) current psychosocial stage of victim (Erikson, 1968); and demographic factors (e.g., age, SES, education, etc.).

As noted earlier, the major debate in the field is over individual vs. trauma factors as necessary and sufficient for causing PTSD. Wilson and Krauss (1985) also note the importance of situational variables. Of crucial importance is where the trauma was experienced (e.g., at home, in familiar surroundings, in a foreign country, etc.).

Environment

Green, Wilson, and Lindy (1985) note that the recovery environment is often neglected in theoretical formulations of PTSD. They argue that the qualities of the environs in which the person attempts to work through the traumatic experience are correlated with outcome. Environmental factors include (1) social supports; (2) protectiveness of family and friends ("trauma membrane"); (3) attitudes of society; (4) intactness of community; and (5) cultural characteristics. With Vietnam veterans and rape victims the recovery environment is often less supportive than it is for disaster victims, the victims of assault or crimes, etc.

Outcome

Two broadly differentiated outcome categories are proposed by Wilson and Krauss (1985). "Pathological outcomes" refer to the development of PTSD, as well as other DSM-III disorders (e.g., psychosis, character pathology, etc.). "Personal growth and restabilization" result with full working through of the trauma. Wilson and Krauss (1985) note that "restabilization indicates that a nonpathological integration of the experience has occurred even though the individual may manifest some symptoms that are dynamically connected to traumatic events (e.g., hypervigilance, occasional nightmares, positive character changes, etc.)" (p. 108).

Summary

The psychosocial model of PTSD is a general model applicable to all traumatic experiences. The research conducted by Wilson and Krauss (1985) with Vietnam combat veterans supports the central assumptions of the model. In particular, correlations were confirmed between degree/nature of trauma and severity of PTSD, the lack of social support and severity of PTSD, and the lack of significance between premorbid personality factors and the development of PTSD. The best predictors of PTSD were the severity of the stressor and the degree of psychosocial isolation in the recovery environment. "If exposure to traumatic stressors in combat lays the foundation for potential changes in the personality structure of the survivor, then the recovery environment may determine whether or not the post-trauma adaptation is pathological or positive in nature" (p. 144).

A BEHAVIORAL (LEARNING THEORY) FORMULATION

Given the evidence pointing to the behavioral treatment of PTSD as the treatment of choice for traumatic stress reactions (see below, Chapter 8: Behavioral Treatment), the understanding of PTSD from a behavioral/ learning theory perspective is crucial. Keane, Zimering, and Caddell (1985) have provided the most comprehensive behavioral formulation of PTSD to date.

Keane et al. (1985) posit a "two factor learning theory of psychopathology" to account for the acquisition and maintenance of PTSD. It is applicable to all patient populations manifesting PTSD.

> Originally postulated by Mowrer (1947; 1960), two factor theory states that psychopathology is a function of both (a) classical conditioning, wherein a fear response is learned through associative principles, and (b) instrumental learning whereby individuals will avoid those conditioned cues that evoke anxiety. (pp. 9–10)

It is, in essence, Stampfl and Levis's (1967; Levis & Hare, 1977; Levis & Boyd, 1979) adaptation of Mowrer's (1947, 1960) theory which is employed by Keane et al. (1985) to explain PTSD. Keane et al. (1985) note the complexity of PTSD symptomatology. Several concepts must be used to account for the different phenomena.

Conditioning of Cues

A cue is a signal. It determines when and where a person responds. It also determines which response to make (Dollard & Miller, 1950). A cue can be an external event. For example, the sound of thunder can be a cue to organize a person to do the behaviors associated with raining. However, cues can also be thoughts, particular people, specific times, and so on. Furthermore, cues can become organized into clusters, so that the specific combination of cues will determine the response. This is called patterning (Dollard & Miller, 1950). For example, darkness alone may not cause a rape victim to become afraid. It may take a combination of darkness, walking on a deserted street, and hearing footsteps to trigger the fear response.

Stimulus Generalization

"Stimulus generalization proposes that the more similar a novel stimulus is to a conditioned stimulus, the stronger the responses will be to that stimulus (Keane et al., 1985, p.10). Hence, a loud noise may be similar enough to the sound of gunfire to evoke a dramatic response in a Vietnam veteran with combat-related PTSD. Generalization can occur based on the simple similarity of two stimuli. It can also occur in a different manner that is quite relevant to PTSD. If two cues or cue patterns are given the same verbal label, the degree of generalization increases (Dollard & Miller, 1950). For instance, the verbal label of "danger" is usually applied to a traumatic situation. If any other cue is given the label of "danger" the fear response of the "dangerous" traumatic situation has an increased probability of generalizing to the new "dangerous" cue.

Higher-Order Conditioning

Once a cue has been conditioned to elicit fear, it in itself will become fearful. Therefore, any cue that consistently precedes the conditioned cue will also be able to elicit the same fear reaction (Dollard & Miller, 1950). Keane et al. (1985) posit that higher-order conditioning is involved in the complexity of PTSD symptomatology. For example, a man is fighting with his wife while they are driving. In the middle of the argument, an accident occurs. Anger and fighting become cues for the fear, because the man was angry with his wife at the time of the accident. Among other symptoms, the man develops anxiety attacks every Tuesday and Friday afternoon just before the executive meetings. There does not appear to be any direct connection between the meeting and the accident. However, it turns out that in this meeting fighting and anger invariably emerge.

Negative Reinforcement

The experience of trauma and its sequelae are generally aversive. According to the principles of negative reinforcement (NR), behavior that leads to a reduction in an aversive is reinforced and is likely to be repeated. NR can account for many of the associated features of PTSD (Keane et al., 1985). All of the avoidance behaviors and psychic numbing are mediated by NR. Behavioral disturbances such as anger and aggression, drug and alcohol abuse "are conceptualized as behavioral patterns that are functionally reinforced by their capacity to reduce aversive feelings" (Keane et al., 1985 p. 267).

Incomplete Exposure to Memories

To explain the fact that constant exposure to conditioned stimuli does not lead to the extinction of conditioned reponses, Keane et al. (1985) propose that the conditioned stimuli match only part of the traumatic memory constellation; only repeated exposure to stimuli matching the original trauma in its entirety could lead to extinction of resulting symptoms. Further, patients with PTSD actively avoid any possible complete exposure to stimuli resembling the original trauma, including the avoidance of thoughts associated with the trauma. This avoidance may also be reinforced by familial or cultural expectations for the patient not to discuss the trauma. Finally, Keane at al. (1985) hypothesize "state dependent retention" which interferes with memory recall. This refers to the difference between the cognitive/physiological state during which the memory was stored and the state during which recall is sought. Without specific clues an impoverished recall of information results. This incomplete exposure to memories leads to a continuing symptomatic picture.

Summary

In sum, classical conditioning and instrumental learning are used to explain the development of the basic pattern of PTSD. Conditioning of cues, stimulus generalization, higher-order conditioning and incomplete exposure to traumatic memories help explain the complexity of the symptomatology. To borrow an analogy from computers, the learning theory formulation of PTSD can be likened to binary assembly language. It allows the very specific tracking of each stimulus, cue, and response. Therefore, very specific behavioral interventions can be utilized to help "reprogram" the patient. In addition, the more massive the trauma the more likely the individual will be affected at the binary level of functioning.

The potential problem with the behavioral model is that there is the possibility of not paying enough attention to higher-order constructs, such as attribution, motivation, development, and the therapeutic relationship. In practice, just as most computer programmers use more advanced languages than assembly, most clinicians combine behavioral and cognitive therapies. And, while there is not a great deal of discussion about the therapeutic relationship and developmental factors in behavioral discourse, astute clinicians certainly take them into account.

COGNITIVE APPRAISAL MODELS

Two authors, Janoff-Bulman (1985) and Epstein (1990), focus on assumptive constructs that each of us make about the world. Traumatic events are viewed as potent disrupters of these basic assumptions about the self and the world. PTSD is viewed as maladaptive coping responses to the invalidation of these basic beliefs (depicted in Table 6.1)

According to Epstein (1990), "everyone unwittingly constructs a personal theory of reality that contains subdivisions of a self theory and a world theory. A personal theory of reality has four basic functions:

- To maintain a favorable pleasure-pain balance over the foreseeable future
- To assimilate the data of reality in a manner that can be coped with
- To maintain a favorable level of self-esteem. (p. 2)
- The need for relatedness (the need to relate to other people)

An individual's personal theory of reality changes and grows through the interaction of assimilation and accommodation. Generally, this process proceeds without a problem. However, in the case of severe trauma the victim may be unable to assimilate the experience into the old personal theory of reality. Some degree of intrusive thoughts and anxiety are viewed as natural and healthy responses. They occur until the maximum amount of information has been assimilated and appropriate accommodation has occurred.

PTSD is "produced by a threatening event that invalidates at a deep experiential level, the three most fundamental beliefs in a personal

Table 6.1. Comparison of Janoff-Bulman's Assumptions and Epstein's Beliefs

Janoff-Bulman's three basic assumptions	Epstein's three fundamental beliefs in a personal theory of reality
1. The belief in personal invulnerability	1. The world is benevolent and a source of joy
2. The perception of the world as meaningful and comprehensible	2. The world is meaningful and controllable
3. The view of the self in a positive light (p. 18)	3. The self is worthy (e.g., lovable, good, and competent)

theory of reality.…The three beliefs concern the degree to which the world is viewed as benevolent and a source of joy; as meaningful and comprehensible (which includes predictable, controllable and just); and the self as worthy (which includes loveable, good and competent)." (p. 3)

Janoff-Bulman (1985) proposed that PTSD following victimization (e.g. rape, muggings, car accidents) is largely a function of the shattering of basic assumptions that the victims had held about themselves and the world. She identifies three basic assumptions that are shared by most people that are usually affected. These assumptions are (1) the belief in personal invulnerability; (2) the perception of the world as meaningful and comprehensible; and (3) the view of ourselves in a positive light. (p. 18)

The Assumption of Invulnerability

Let us consider for a minute the assumption that "it can't happen to me." We all assume that when we are driving *no one* will cross the double yellow line. Or consider for a moment the famous shower scene from Hitchcock's *Psycho*. Most of us would think, "That could never really happen." It just so happens that one of the authors was home alone, taking a shower and shampooing his hair. He heard a noise, and jokingly thought to himself, "Ha ha ha, *Psycho*." He heard the noise again, and thought the same thought. He heard the noise a third time. This time he was concerned. When he opened the shower door, there was a strange person in the bathroom! Luckily, nothing came of this. It was not a rape, or a mugging or floor collapsing. In this situation there was no bodily damage. The lack of dangerousness was assessed within a few seconds. However, the assumption that strange people only enter bathrooms in movies was effectively shattered. Nevertheless, it took two years for him to be able to close his eyes while shampooing his hair alone in the house without anxiety.

People who have been victimized can no longer think, "It can't happen to me." There is a marked sense of vulnerability, and the fear that if it can happen once, the same victimization can happen again (Janoff-Bulman, 1985). The effect of altering the assumption of invulnerability becomes acutely clear in the finding that rape victims who experienced serious physical injury or the *cognitive appraisal of life threat* were almost three times more likely to have developed PTSD than rape victims who did not experience serious physical injury or the *cognitive appraisal of life threat!* (Kilpatrick et al., 1989).

The change from regarding oneself as invulnerable to regarding oneself as vulnerable corresponds to the change of belief that the world is benign to the belief that it is malevolent (Epstein, 1989).

The World as Meaningful

Janoff-Bulman (1985) points out that according to prior research people generally regard their world as controllable, predictable, and just. The victimization invalidates this assumption and forces individuals to search for new meanings and assumptions about the world and themselves to fit in with the new personal experience. The central question for a victim is not, "Why do these terrible events happen?" Rather, it is, "Why did this happen to me (or a significant other)?" (Janoff-Bulman, 1985). Unfortunately, there generally are not any "good, logical" answers. The result is that until equilibrium is reestablished the world for the victim is not meaningful nor is it controllable or predictable. In one large study of victimization (Kilpatrick, personal communication, March 1988) symptom severity (as measured by the SCL-90) had a negative correlation of .80 with a measure of victim satisfaction with the justice system! In other words, the more the victim felt a lack of support by the agencies of justice (which would tend to invalidate an assumption of a just and meaningful world), the more severe were the victim's symptoms. The potential problem is that the need for meaning may force the victim into regressive irrational modes of thinking in order to find an answer.

The Self as Worthy

People attempt to maintain a favorable level of self-esteem (Epstein, 1989), and operate under the assumption that they are decent people who do not deserve to be victimized (Janoff-Bulman, 1985). However, once they have been victimized there are numerous sources that undermine a sense of self-worth. These include:

- a sense of helplessness about the victimization
- further confusion and helplessness about the uncontrollable thoughts and feelings in reaction to the event (e.g. weakness, fearfulness, intrusive thoughts and imagery)
- reasonable or unreasonable demands of the self to have been able to do more to prevent the event or to help others (e.g., in an accident)
- diminished sense of competence

In support of his theory Epstein (1989) presents data from the factor analytic study of symptoms in Vietnam veterans by Wilson and Krause (1985). The largest factor of this factor analysis provides strong support for the three basic beliefs in a personal theory of reality. The factor had four clusters. The first cluster refers to a loss of meaning. The second cluster corresponds to loss of self-esteem. The third group of items relates to an unfavorable pleasure-pain balance. Finally, the fourth cluster pointed to the significant disturbance in the PTSD veterans degree of relatedness with others. It is interesting to note that of the 7 factors that were discerned the largest factor (18%) was existential in nature, whereas the next largest factor (11%) was anxiety; and intrusive imagery accounted for only 7% of the variance: thereby lending support to the view of the psychosocial nature of the disorder.

Summary

The cognitive appraisal model of PTSD emphasizes the importance of individuals' basic assumptions and beliefs about the self and the world that usually are not seriously challenged at a deep level. Traumatic events have the potential to shatter these basic assumptions. While some form of post-traumatic response is seen as healthy, PTSD is viewed as maladaptive coping responses to the invalidation of these basic beliefs.

The model has several advantages. There is growing empirical support for the importance of cognitive appraisal in trauma (Epstein, 1989; Kilpatrick et al., 1989). The model allows for a continuum of normal to pathological responses to trauma. The relevance of broken assumptions and fragmented personal theories of the self and the world corresponds to the experiential realities of people with PTSD. The emphasis on cognitive appraisal of the role of the self points to specific possibilities for therapeutic intervention.

The cognitive appraisal model has the added benefit of being highly compatible or complementary with other views of PTSD. The emphasis on how an individual derives meaning about the self and the world is congruent with many of the ideas in the psychodynamic approaches. The role of environmental response is important, because it will effect how the individual appraises "the world."

A PSYCHODYNAMIC ("CLASSICAL") FORMULATION

Historically psychoanalytic theories have been used to explain the combat neuroses of soldiers (e.g., Freud, 1919; Kardiner, 1941) and the traumatic neuroses of holocaust survivors (e.g., Krystal, 1968). Although the majority of psychoanalytic writers have theorized that genetic factors are the most predictive of PTSD (e.g., Grinker & Speigal, 1945), Rappaport (1968) notes that there has been some recognition in the psychoanalytic community of the importance of the traumatic experience itself. This position is supported by Niederland (1968), who notes:

> The etiology of these conditions has all too frequently been attributed to the *Anlage,* the constitution, to other events, endogenous factors, or to the abuse or misuse of psychoanalytic concepts, to something that went on between the survivors and their parents during the first and second years of life. (p. 63)

Thus, Rappaport (1968) sees the need for a revision of the traditional understanding of neurosis with respect to extreme traumatization. However, much psychoanalytic and psychoanalytically informed thinking about PTSD continues to place a major emphasis upon the constitution of the individual and the various pre-trauma conflicts in the psyche (e.g., Worthington, 1978). This is particularly true in "informal settings" (e.g., community mental health clinics) where it is the individual's weaknesses which are seen as the "cause" of PTSD, rather than the nature and extent of the stress. [Hence, classical psychoanalytic literature dealing with traumatic stress is often characterized as having individual focus, and criticized for ignoring the realities of war, concentration camps, rape, assault, disaster, etc. (Williams, 1980b).]

What a classical psychoanalytic perspective can offer is a greater understanding of the reaction of the individual's psyche to traumatic stress. Hendin et al. (1981) using several cases of combat-related PTSD, describe the interaction between early childhood learnings and attitudes and the actual circumstances of the wartime stressors. As a function of the interaction of these factors, each veteran developed specific meanings to their combat experience, that were relevant to their specific presentation.

Grubrich-Simitis (1981) outlines a psychoanalytic understanding of the effects of extreme traumatization with reference to the survivors of concentration camps during World War II. It is one of the clearest expositions of victims' responses in terms of classical psychoanalytic ideas. Although the nature of the stressors is acknowledged, there is an emphasis on the pre-traumatic personality and the pre-morbid capacity to tolerate stress as having a significant bearing on the development of psychopathology. Grubrich-Simitis (1981) notes the importance of the following stressors:

- disruption of family ties/loss of sociocultural environment
- witnessing atrocities
- continuous separation anxiety
- perpetual helplessness/anticipation of one's own death
- "barbaric reinfantalization"
- "annihilation of individuality"
- elimination of privacy
- "systematic abrogation of the principle of causality"
- constant debasement/degradation.

The consequences of the above is that "where ego was, id shall be." Primary needs thus become paramount and rule all behavior. From a classically oriented psychoanalytic perspective the following occur as a consequence:

- a drive regression to orality
- a displacement of libidinal cathexis from object to self representations (especially body image)
- progressive drive defusion
- remobilization of infantile sado-masochistic drive impulses
- regressive changes in ego (especially defensive organization)
- denial became primary defense
- development of a "false self"/"automatization of the ego"/
- "robotization"
- identification with the aggressor
- regression to archaic forms of superego functioning
- destructive changes in ego ideal

Grubrich-Simitis (1981) notes that the aforementioned alterations in psychic functioning were necessary for survival. However, they also resulted in "irreversible structural damage" to the psyche. Most notable are:

- a fragile ego structure
- chronic continuous use of denial
- escape into an inner world of memories/fantasies

- hypochondriasis (from libidinization of body)
- impaired interpersonal functioning (from ego-automatization)
- avoidance of cathexis to new objects
- maintenance of cathexis to old/lost objects
- constant alertness (fearfulness of repetition)
- severe pathology of aggressive drives resulting in depression, guilt, paranoia, turning against the self, projection, and somatization
- possible asocial characteristics (from infiltration of enemy-image into superego and ego ideal)
- shattered basic trust

Grubrich-Simitis (1981) stresses the intractable nature of the changes brought about by extreme traumatization, and notes the difficulties many (psychoanalytic) therapists have had treating the survivors of concentration camps. Rappaport (1968) echoes this concern, noting, "...the regenerative powers of the ego are not limitless...the human spirit can be broken beyond repair, [and] the damage can go "beyond" a traumatic neurosis, a term which can almost sound like a euphemism" (p. 730).

Summary

The classical psychoanalytic position has frequently overemphasized the pre-trauma personality as the major factor in determining the possible development of PTSD after trauma. Current data, strongly refutes this assertion. Certainly, classical analytic treatment is not the treatment of choice for PTSD. Nevertheless, the roles of conflict, regression (especially in ego functioning), transference and countertransference can provide greater understanding of the reaction of the individual's psyche to traumatic stress, as well as the nuances of the therapeutic relationship.

A PSYCHOSOCIAL-DEVELOPMENTAL (ERIKSON)/ PSYCHOFORMATIVE (LIFTON) MODEL

Drawing upon the theories of Erikson (1946, 1968) and Lifton (1967, 1973, 1976), Wilson (1977, 1978) has suggested a psychosocial model which highlights the effects of massive trauma on development. Although this model was constructed with specific reference to Vietnam veterans, it is applicable to other patient populations. Indeed, Wilson's (1977, 1978) focus on Erikson's (1968) fifth psychosocial stage, the stage at which most soldiers went to Vietnam, adds to observations that the impact of extreme traumatization is most disruptive to those in adolescence and early adulthood. Although this model is not a model of PTSD exclusively, it accounts for many of the observations made of patients manifesting PTSD since all PTSD patients have experienced extreme traumatization.

A Psychosocial-Developmental Perspective

Erikson's (1968) model of development and ego identity is epigenetic in nature. It posits a universal sequence of psychosocial stages and incorporates the interaction of the person's genetic makeup and extraindividual influences upon growth. Each psychosocial stage is conceived of as a "crisis" or "transition," and thus each stage has a "task." The resolution of each stage has profound effects upon the resulting personal identity.

Wilson (1977) highlights the fifth psychosocial crisis: identity vs. role confusion. He notes:

> This developmental period has as its "task" the need to assume the various roles of adulthood and to meet adequately the demands that accompany them. This crisis is especially important since the doubts, uncertainties, insecurities, as well as personal and social competencies of a person, must be interwoven into a more coherent and enduring sense of self that links the historical past in continuity with the present. (p. 6)

Echoing Erikson (1968), Wilson (1980) emphasizes the importance of this stage in the formation of a sense of wholeness and identity. Most cultures provide a "psychosocial moratorium" during this phase of growth to allow the late adolescent/young adult the opportunity to explore and to consolidate the identity.

When the psychosocial moratorium is disrupted, the ability of the individual to attend to the task of his/her psychosocial stage is interfered with. The result is "role confusion" or "identity confusion." Other features of a disrupted psychosocial moratorium in phase V include:

- confusion over the future
- the sense that time is unmanageable, fleeting, uncontrollable
- fears that aspects of one's behavior are uncontrollable
- self-consciousness
- sense of being "fixed" into roles
- frustration associated with the inability to reach goals
- the avoidance of intimate relationships
- strong anxiety
- a sense of alienation
- disruption in ideology (i.e., value formation)

Wilson (1978) notes that many of the above sequelae of a disrupted psychosocial moratorium are characteristic of Vietnam combat veterans. Those unable to reach a balance, to complete the psychosocial task, struggle to find meaning and purpose in their lives. "Psychic numbing" is common in those most affected (e.g., PTSD populations).

Wilson (1978) extends this psychosocial perspective beyond the fifth stage to include the "post-identity" stages. Put otherwise, his focus is on the effects of a disrupted psychosocial moratorium on the entire sequence of subsequent psychosocial stages. He notes that most Vietnam veterans are currently in the sixth psychosocial stage (intimacy vs. isolation). Since epigenesis implies that the resolution of the preceding crisis affects the ability to resolve future psychosocial crises, it is hypothesized that difficulties will be manifested in the ability to resolve the intimacy vs. isolation task. Not surprisingly, a strong sense of identity and self-esteem are required to constructively engage in intimate relationships.

With respect to many Vietnam veterans, the sixth psychosocial stage was resolved in the direction of isolation rather than intimacy. Wilson (1978) attributes this to a disrupted psychosocial moratorium and the unsupportive environment the veterans returned to which contributed to the difficulties in crisis resolution.

Wilson (1978) also looks ahead to the crises of generativity vs. stagnation (the seventh psychosocial stage) and integrity vs. despair (the last psychosocial stage). The inability to resolve preceding tasks will, Wilson (1978) hypothesizes, make it more difficult to resolve future developmental tasks. An inability to form intimate bonds results in isolation and "distantiation" (Erikson, 1968). "Distantiation or isolation refers to the estrangement created by withdrawal from attempts to fuse ego boundaries" (Wilson, 1978, p. 9). Hence, the individual fears loss of identity/self-esteem, fears rejection, prematurely rejects others to avoid pain, or may experience sexual confusion.

Wilson (1978) notes that one of the most difficult problems for returning veterans was, and is, the ability to successfully navigate intimate relationships. He notes a "purposeful distantiation" on the part of veterans associated with the distantiation fostered in combat (i.e., "If I don't get close, I don't have to suffer the loss [of my good buddy; of myself]").

The final stage of psychosocial development raises the issues of death and the existential meaning of life. Wilson (1978) hypothesizes that veterans will engage in a reprocessing of their wartime experiences. Successful navigation of this stage promotes a sense of integrity; failure to resolve the crisis of the final stage results in despair.

A PSYCHOFORMATIVE PERSPECTIVE

As noted above, Wilson (1978) also draws on the theories of Lifton (1967, 1976, 1979). Wilson (1978) summarizes the psychoformative perspective as follows:

> The controlling image or paradigm in Lifton's work centers around death and the continuity of life. The core constructs of his thinking are concerned with how individuals change, transform, and evolve formative symbols (images and forms) in the process of experience which has as anchor points death and life (p. 17).

Within psychoformative theory are three "subparadigms." These represent basic formative modes of thinking/symbolizing:

- connection (i.e., the sense of "connectedness") vs. separation (i.e., the idea of death)
- integrity (i.e., intact physical/ego boundaries) vs. disintegration (i.e., threat to organismic intactness)
- movement (i.e., development, progress, change) vs. stasis (i.e., cessation of growth, autonomy, wholeness, etc.)

Each pole of these three subparadigms has its own associated images.

The sense of vitality and aliveness is associated with connection, integrity, and movement. A person who feels this way feels "centered." However, with trauma, "uncentering" may occur and "...the person will not be able to assimilate the new experience into pre-existing psychoformative modes of being" (Wilson, 1978, p. 20). "Grounding" refers to the ability of the person to "decenter" without "uncentering" (i.e., "recentering" is possible). When the processes of centering and grounding are impaired, "psychic numbing" results. This includes (Lifton, 1976) (1) An inability to feel; (2) gaps between knowledge and feelings; (3) apathy and "deadening;" anger/rage; and (4) impairment of psychoformative processes.

Psychic numbing thus constellates the separation, disintegration, and stasis poles of the three subparadigms. Further, the person is uncentered and lacks the ability to recenter.

A Combined Psychosocial and Psychoformative Perspective

In his analysis of the effects of the Vietnam war on persons in the fifth psychosocial stage of development, Wilson (1978) integrates the perspectives of Erikson (1968) and Lifton (1976). He is particularly interested in the effect of trauma on the developing personality. Wilson (1978, 1980; Wilson & Krauss, 1985) notes that as a consequence of trauma the ego may undergo:

• retrogression to earlier modes of psychosocial adaptation
• psychosocial acceleration (i.e., new ego strengths and capacities emerge prematurely);
• exacerbation of current psychosocial stages, thus intensifying the experience/conflict of that stage; and
• a change in hierarchical arrangements of needs (e.g., the need for safety or power may become salient).

Although psychosocial acceleration has been noted, more frequently, "The intensity of the war experiences seems to have stressed psychosocial and psychoformative processes beyond an optimal level" (Wilson, 1978, p. 27). Indeed, the effect of trauma often has the effect of negatively constellating the "negative" poles of both Erikson's (1968) psychosocial stages (including those already transited [through regression], and those to be faced) and Lifton's (1976) psychoformative subparadigms. Clearly these characteristics refer in large measure to the personality constructs of PTSD patients.

With specific reference to psychic numbing, Wilson (1978) notes that psychosocial attributes include acute identity diffusion, mistrust, doubt, feelings of inferiority, work paralysis, despair, stagnation, isolation, and withdrawal. Psychoformative processes are characterized by blockage of processes, a strong sense of uncentering, stasis, separation, and disintegration. The belief system of those with psychic numbing includes ideological confusion and a confusion of values. Finally, affective motivational components of psychic numbing include feelings of hopelessness/helplessness, rage, anger, guilt, depression, low self-esteem, anxiety, etc.

Summary

Wilson's (1977, 1978, 1980; Wilson & Krauss, 1985) model of the effects of trauma on the developing personality integrates the theoretical orientations of Erikson (1968) and Lifton (1976). In essence, Wilson (1978) examines the effects of trauma and the disruption of the psychosocial moratorium during the fifth psychosocial stage on the development of ego identity. In addition, he notes the characteristic psychoformative features resulting from trauma. Although this model was devised with reference to Vietnam veterans in general, there is a clear focus on those veterans who were traumatized (and thus had a high chance of developing PTSD). Also, since the effects of trauma on late adolescents/early adults has been regarded as particularly damaging, the theories suggested may also help understand victims of other forms of extreme traumatization.

AN OBJECT RELATIONS THEORY FORMULATION

In his studies of PTSD, Brende (1982, 1983) notes the similarities in Vietnam veteran character pathology to various disorders of self (i.e., borderline and narcissistic personality disorders). Although his theorizing is restricted to the Vietnam combat veteran population, the "splitting" of the personality in response to severe trauma may be extended to other patient groups with PTSD. The theoretical perspectives underlying Brende's (1983) hypotheses are drawn from American Object Relations theorists (e.g., Mahler et al., 1975; Masterson, 1976; Rinsley, 1982; Kernberg, 1975; Kohut, 1971).

Characteristics found in both Vietnam veteran PTSD patients and patients manifesting borderline and/or narcissistic character pathology include: self-defeating behavior, idealization and devaluation, outbursts of uncontrollable rage, identity diffusion, abandonment, depression, impaired emotional responsiveness, utilization of primitive defenses (e.g., splitting, denial, projective identification), a sense of meaninglessness.

Brende (1983) posits that the varied and pronounced stressors experienced by certain groups of Vietnam veterans had a fragmenting effect on identity. The result is a loss of identity, the development of "splits" in the self-system, pathological killer-victim identifications, omnipotence, and the emergence of a "protective self."

Loss of Self-Identity

Brende (1983) notes that the degree and permanency of character change differs between combat veterans of World War II and of the Vietnam confrontation. The more protracted identity difficulties are attributed to differences in pre-combat training and wartime experience. The result is a post-traumatic loss of the sense of self characterized by emotional detachment.

Splits in the Self-System

Brende (1983) notes that object relations theorists have pointed to splits in the self-system resulting in the failure of the separation-individuation process (Mahler et al., 1975; Masterson & Rinsley, 1975). The result is an "idealized part-self object" and a "devalued part-self object" (Kernberg, 1975). Brende (1983) argues that departure from the "mother country" to the dangers of Vietnam represented a destructive recapitulation of the separation-individuation process for Vietnam recruits. The "mother country" was unsupportive and unavailable; the ineffective military and detached political leaders (i.e., "fathers") betrayed the ideals of recruits and failed to serve as role models for gender identification; helplessness was axiomatic; aggression was not healthily integrated and utilized for the separation-individuation project. In sum, the experience of abandonment and betrayal led to the failure of normal separation-individuation and identity consolidation. In addition, "The self became realigned and polarized into "good" (idealized) and "bad" (devalued) aspects" (Brende, 1983, p. 202). Values became distorted, emotional expression was devalued, and aggression became idealized.

Pathological Killer-Identification: The Killer-Self

Wilson (1980) argues that the disruptions in veterans' lives occurred during the fifth developmental phase of identity formation (Erikson, 1968). Hence, the crisis of identity vs. role confusion was salient during the Vietnam era for most veterans. Brende (1983) notes:

> The attempt by many American soldiers to consolidate an idealized mental construct of "being a man" during military training often led to a pathological, idealizing identification with an aggressor, with the ensuing development of a "killer" identity. (p. 203)

Combat experiences often consolidated the identification with the aggressor. Hence the "killer self."

Pathological Victim Identification: The Victim-Self

Brende (1983) notes that victims of traumatic events often become self-destructive, either overtly or through somatization. The "helpless" part (of the "bad self") manifests "...the persistent symptoms of vague anxiety, unpleasant memories, nightmares, headaches, dizzy spells, and pains in his body" (Brende & Benedict, 1980). In essence, the victims of the veteran's killer-self are introjected and become part of the self-system. Hence, the emergence of a "victim self."

Pathological Omnipotence

Brende (1983) argues that pathological omnipotence emerges as a defense against awareness of the victim-self. Aggression and/or risk-taking behavior are also employed to maintain repression of this aspect of the personality.

The Protective Self

In addition to defensive aggressive omnipotence, Brende (1985) argues that a "protective self" also emerges. This idealized part-self identification is structurally equivalent to the self-object underlying narcissism in both borderline and narcissistic personality disorders. Brende (1985) notes that the protective self emerges for survivor purposes. It emerged amidst symbiotic relationships within the combat unit, and included the introjection of the other members to such an extent that the loss of "buddies" was felt as a loss of part of the self. The result was often psychotic-like rage reactions. Aggressively protective behavior is also associated with the need to maintain split-off feelings of helplessness, guilt, grief, and fear, primarily through denial.

Summary

Brende's (1983, 1985) Object Relations Theory model of PTSD rests upon the power of the trauma to effect "splits" in the personality. With Vietnam combat veterans such splits bring about characteristic part-self identifications, defenses, and a pathologically constellated identity. Certainly the impact of other massive traumas may have a similar effect on the psyches of potential victims, and thus the model has applicability beyond the Vietnam combat veteran population.

The emphasis on splits in the personality complements several other models of pathology such as Watkin & Watkin's (1981) ego-state model and Hilgard's (1974) neo-dissociation models of cognition. All of these models express the importance of dissociative quality of PTSD that was reflected in the debate by the DSM-III-R committee on PTSD to place the diagnosis with the dissociative disorders.

The model can add some depth to the understanding of certain individuals and the disorder in general. It also offers an interesting rationale for patients to experience many of the dysphoric feelings they are likely to experience, namely to reintegrate the parts of themselves that they have split off. The potential problem with this type of model is that there can be a tendency to reify the descriptions. It also does not account for the many environmental factors that influence the development of PTSD.

PSYCHOPHYSIOLOGIC/PSYCHOBIOLOGIC MODELS

Two models have been posited to explain PTSD from a psychophysiologic/psychobiologic perspective. De la Pena (1984) suggests a brain-modulated, compensatory information-augmenting response in individuals characterized by low levels of central nervous system (CNS) information flow. Van der Kolk et al. (1984) and van der Kolk and Greenberg (1987) propose that PTSD is a biologically based disorder.

PTSD as a Brain-Modulated, Compensatory Information-Augmenting Response

De la Pena (1984) has outlined a psychophysiologic model PTSD etiology as it pertains to Vietnam veterans. Various assumptions underlie this model:

- The nervous system is an "information processing system."
- "Level of arousal" is related to the rate of information processing in subsystems.
- An "overall information processing rate" characterizes the CNS.
- The above is "highly correlated with the 'sum' of the information processing rated in the various hierarchically organized information subsystems." (p. 113)

De la Pena (1984) posits that "parasympathetic-dominant" individuals (PDI) have a higher risk of developing PTSD than others. Such individuals ordinarily experience a lower rate of information flow in the CNS when exposed to a normal level of sensory stimuli than "sympathetic-dominant individuals" (SDI). Apparently PDI habituate more quickly to sensory information. The result is an attempt by the brain to augment its own information flow to enhance perceptive, behavioral, and behavioral functioning.

In combat situations the PDI is more able to tolerate the uncertainty and increased information load. Instead of experiencing boredom (i.e., information underload), the PDI now experiences an optimal level of psychophysiologic functioning. De la Pena (1984) describes the combat situation as "information-rich." The result is interest and feelings of relaxation. Also, cortical structures develop to handle the increased information flow, and the PDI develops a preferred rate of information flow above his/her constitutionally set level. However, when the PDI is no longer in an environment with a high information flow, there is a "rebound." CNS information flow drops steeply to "aberrantly low levels." Hence, in ordinary sensory environments the PDI veteran experiences something akin to sensory deprivation and severe boredom and depression.

Given the experience of a preferred rate of information flow during combat, the veteran in noncombat situations attempts to augment the information flow. De la Pena (1984) argues that this explains many of the common symptoms of PTSD: nightmares, insomnia, hypervigilance, impulsive (excitement seeking) behaviors, aggressive outbursts, etc. Hence, many PTSD symptoms are

> posited to be the expression of maladaptive information-augmenting mechanisms by which the understimulated, bored brain attempts to rectify its aberrantly low information flow rates to higher, more intermediate levels associated with organized perceptual-cognitive-behavioral function and the experience of interest. (p. 117)

De la Pena (1984) supports the above by noting the tendency for PTSD veterans to fall into REM periods more quickly than SDI. He hypothesizes that the information-rich REM periods are part of the brain's attempt to increase information flow.

PTSD as a Biologically Based Disorder

Van der Kolk et al. (1984) and van der Kolk and Greenberg (1987) build upon the learned helplessness model developed by Maier & Seligman (1967). They note that in animals, norepinephrine (NE) turnover increases with exposure to inescapable shock. The result is:

- increased levels of plasma catecholamine levels
- decreased levels of brain NE
- increased production of 3-methoxy-4-hydroxphenylglycol (MHPG)
- decreased levels of brain dopamine (DA)
- decreased levels of brain seratonin
- increased levels of acetylcholine
- an analgesic response, mediate by endogenous opioids

NE depletion is correlated with a deficiency of escape behavior, and DA depletion results in a decreased capacity for the animal to initiate a response. Repeated exposure to inescapable shock leads to analgesia, with the development of analgesia as a conditioned response to even mild stressors.

Eventually an "addiction to the trauma" can occur. Van der Kolk et al. (1984) note the tendency for victims of trauma to seek out stimuli not unlike the original experience. They note that traumatic exposure leads to a CNS opioid response. Opioids, including endogenous opioid peptides, have the following psychoactive properties: (1) tranquilizing action; (2) reduction of rage/aggression; (3) reduction of paranoia; (4) reduction of feelings of inadequacy; and (5) antidepressant actions. Van der Kolk et al. (1984) also note the similarities between opioid withdrawal and the PTSD symptoms.

Hence, van der Kolk et al. (1984) posit that the initiation and maintenance of PTSD and post-traumatic states are mediated by the central noradrenergic system and CNS opioid peptides. Reexposure to traumatic situations thus enhances opioid production and brings a sense of control. When the stressor terminates, the individual goes through opioid withdrawl.

Summary

De la Pena (1984) hypothesizes a constitutionally based factor which explains the predisposition of some individuals for developing PTSD. He argues that this model explains the paradoxical clinical finding that Vietnam veterans with PTSD frequently become more relaxed with stimulants, and more anxious with depressants. Clearly the stimulants return information flow to preferred levels, whereas depressants lower an already low level of information flow. Van der Kolk et al. (1984) and van der Kolk and Greenberg (1987) propose altered brain physiology as both an initiating and maintenance factor in PTSD.

The main danger of biological models, from our perspective, is that they are often used to search for the magic pill. These models offer several interesting possibilities. First, particularly difficult cases may have symptoms that are strongly under biological control. Appropriate psychopharmacological intervention can then be used adjunctively (see Chapter 15). Second, behavioral interventions may be designed on the basis of these models. For example, based on the addiction to trauma model (Van der Kolk & Greenberg, 1987) a behavioral prescription of running may aid the person in switching triggers for endogenous opioid production from rage attacks.

A CYBERNETIC MODEL

Schultz (1984) proposes a cybernetic model for PTSD which builds upon prevailing psychodynamic and behavioral models of the disorder. Although it is similar to the psychosocial model proposed by Green, Wilson, and Lindy (1985), it adds cybernetic understanding to various interactions and feedback loops.

Schultz (1984) argues that memories of combat lead to increased physiological arousal, and vice versa. Hence, a "deviation-amplifying cybernetic circuit" develops. Following basic cybernetic principles Schultz (1984) argues that this amplification in the circuit continues until the circuit is broken (i.e., the capacity to remember or become aroused reaches a limit, or the feedback is disrupted) or a "higher order mechanism" depresses the feedback loop. Examples of higher-order mechanisms include avoidance, denial, emotional numbing, and depression. Thus, Schultz (1984) sees the cybernetic model as including both the physiological (attended to by behavioral theorists) and psychological dimensions (attended to by psychodynamically oriented theorists).

Schultz (1984) then adds a third dimension to the cybernetic model, the deviation-reducing impact of the social environment. At root, the influence of those around a PTSD patient is to "limit the activity in the original deviation-amplifying circuit." Therapy may also be included in the expanded cybernetic model. Various techniques learned by the patient (e.g., deep breathing for relaxation) also serve to break the original arousal-memories circuit. "This new form of self-regulation is more effective...and replaces the old type of self-regulation (suppressing behaviors) and the social regulation of the post-traumatic symptoms" (p. 453).

Summary

The cybernetic model of PTSD brings systems theory to our understanding of the disorder. Schultz (1984) argues that the causality found in behavioral and psychoanalytic theories is "linear," and thus must postulate ongoing "causes" for the "effects" (e.g., respondent conditioning and the repetition compulsion). In contrast, the cybernetic model introduces "circular" causality. Hence, the persistence of various PTSD symptoms are seen as epiphenomenon of a cybernetic circuit. As long as the circuit remains intact, the symptoms will occur. The effect of symptoms (e.g., outbursts of rage) and medications (e.g., MAO inhibitors) are seen as agents which impact the original cybernetic circuit and affect deviation-reduction.

A cybernetic circuit that leads to a particular individual's PTSD can be simple or complex. The primary goal of treatment is to break the pathological circuit.[7] In a cybernetic framework, treatment difficulty is a function of circuit redundancy. Redundancy occurs when there is more than one to maintain the circuit. For instance, between points A and B there are three wires. Cutting wire 1 will not be sufficient, because the signal is maintained via wires 2 and 3.

The particular advantage of a cybernetic framework is that it allows for multiple causes and multiple solutions. The primary goal is the disruption of the pathological circuit itself. The potential problem with the model is the possibility of becoming lost in the circularity of causation.

There is evidence that some factors are more central than others (e.g. appraisal of danger) in some situations. Given an adequate assessment, it will often be clear that some interventions may have a better possibility of breaking the circuit than others.

SUMMARY: AN ECOSYSTEMIC MODEL

PTSD is a complicated problem. Each of the models has specific advantages and disadvantages. Table 6.2 pairs the symptoms of PTSD with proposed mechanisms from different theoretical orientations.

We feel that it is a mistake to take an either/or position when building a model of PTSD. It is our opinion that a both/and framework is more heuristic.

We have presented the different models of PTSD. However, it is important to have a more integrated understanding of the factors in the development of PTSD. Therefore, we will offer here an integrated model of PTSD that can act as a guide for clinicians. The psychosocial model of Green et al. (1985) is already an integrated model. We will use that as our starting point, and make several additions. Our model is represented visually in Figure 6.2. The asterisks beside certain variables indicates that they are particularly important.

We will elaborate only the ideas that are new or disparate with the psychosocial model.[8] The path towards PTSD is initiated with a traumatic experience. How the person experiences the event is the first factor that will influence the development of PTSD. Some of the variables include: length and intensity of trauma, degree of life threat, bereavement, role of survivor (active vs passive), type of trauma (man-made or natural), the idiosyncratic specifics of the trauma.

The experience of the trauma itself will effect three other variables. The first variable, post-traumatic cognitive processing, follows the psychosocial model (Green et al., 1985). The second variable is that the nature of the trauma itself, as well as the response of the individual will impact on the environment. These variables will influence the environment's response.

For example, the rape of an individual woman, the murder of a child's parents, and a terrorist attack will produce different responses from the environment. On a societal level, women have often been blamed for having done something to provoke the attack. A family or a community may be highly threatened by the "sexual" overtones of a rape. There may be a distancing from the victim. By contrast, there may be an outpouring of community support for children whose parents have been murdered.

The third variable that is influenced by the characteristic of the trauma itself is the degreee of classical conditioning that occurs. The more intense the trauma the more likely a strong conditioned response will occur. The characteristic of the trauma will also influence the type of stimuli that will become conditioned.

An integrated model of PTSD cannot ignore the influences of classical and respondent conditioning. There is a level of nonconscious, nonvolitional response to stimuli and cues that have been conditioned that is essentially automatic. These responses as well as the negatively reinforced avoidance responses influence the intrusion-avoidance gradient (seen in the center of Figure 6.1). For instance, the degree of avoidance behavior in which an individual engages will influence the nature of the information available for processing. The folklore example of getting back on the horse once a person has fallen off is a good metaphor. The person who gets back on has one set of information (e.g., the horse does not always throw you; the anxiety level is not as bad as fantasized, partially due to extinction). The person who does not get on the horse does not have the same information. Furthermore, various cues (e.g. thoughts and images) may become conditioned. For instance, the following sequence can occur. The person thinks the thought, "Perhaps I should try to get back on the horse." Then the rider becomes anxious. If then the individual does not go through with getting on the horse, the thought may become a conditioned cue.

The environment will also effect the reinforcement contingency schedule. The response of the family will effect the person. Does the family reinforce the avoidance and/or the passive role? Does the family differentially support the expression of fear as well as supporting the facing of the feared situation?

The classically conditioned fear responses (such as becoming scared when hearing a loud noise) often become stressors to the individual. They interact with the person's appraisal system, because individuals must make some appraisal of what is happening to them that they are responding this way. The more the person makes self-deprecating appraisals (e. g., "I am going crazy, I must be a weak person") or other deprecating assessments (e.g., "people will laugh at me or think I am crazy"), the more likely the symptoms will become exacerbated. As discussed earlier, cognitive appraisals of the traumatic situation can act as cues (e.g., verbal labels such as "danger").

Green et al. (1985) included cognitive appraisal and meaning under the category of individual chracteristics. We have given the variables of appraisal of meaning a separate category to underscore the importance of these processes. We are following the work of Epstein (1989) and

Table 6.2. PTSD Symptoms and Comparative Mechanisms and Theoretical Orientations

PTSD DSM-III-R symptoms	Mechanisms	Theoretical orientation
B. Reexperiencing the trauma	Assimilation and accommodation	Organismic attempt to make sense of new and traumatic event (Epstein, 1988)
1. Recurrent and intrusive recollections of the event		
2. Recurrent or distressing dreams	Phases of intrusion; failure or relaxation of defensive controls (e.g., ideas and sequences and mental set)	Psychodynamic and information processing (Horowitz, 1986)
3. Sudden acting or feeling as if traumatic event were recurring	Phase of intrusion	Psychodynamic and information processing (Horowitz, 1986)
	Dissociation	None proposed in PTSD literature (Horowitz, [1986] discusses briefly). Relevant discussions are in hypnotic and ego-state literature.
	Addiction to trauma in order to stimulate CNS opioid response that has a tranquilizing action	Psychobiologic model (van der Kolk and Greenberg, 1987)
4. Intense psychological distress at exposure to events that symbolize or resemble the trauma	Generalization of anxiety	Learning theory (classical conditioning)
	Phases of intrusion (symbolic associations)	Psychodynamic and information processing (Horowitz, 1986)

C. Persistent avoidance of stimuli associated with the trauma or numbing of general responsiveness		
1. Deliberate efforts to avoid thoughts or feelings associated with the trauma	Conscious escape behavior and negative reinforcement	Learning theory; operant conditioning
	Phases of denial, use of defensive controls (e.g., ideas and sequences and mental set)	Psychodynamic and information processing (Horowitz, 1986)
2. Deliberate efforts to avoid activities or situations that arouse recollections of trauma	Conscious escape behavior and negative reinforcement	Learning theory; operant conditioning
	Phases of denial, use of defensive controls (e.g., ideas and sequences and mental set)	Psychodynamic and information processing (Horowitz, 1986)
3. Psychogenic amnesia	Generalized avoidance of cues; Dissociation	Dollard & Miller (1950)
4–7. Psychic numbing	Generalized avoidance of cues; Isolation of affect and psychic closing off; Phases of denial	Dollard & Miller (1950); Lifton (1968); Psychodynamic and information processing (Horowitz, 1986)
D. Increased arousal	Stimulus generalization	Learning theory; classical conditioning
	Alteration in CNS functioning influencing autonomic functioning	Psychobiological theories (De la Pena, 1984; van der Kolk et al., 1984; van der Kolk & Greenberg, 1987)

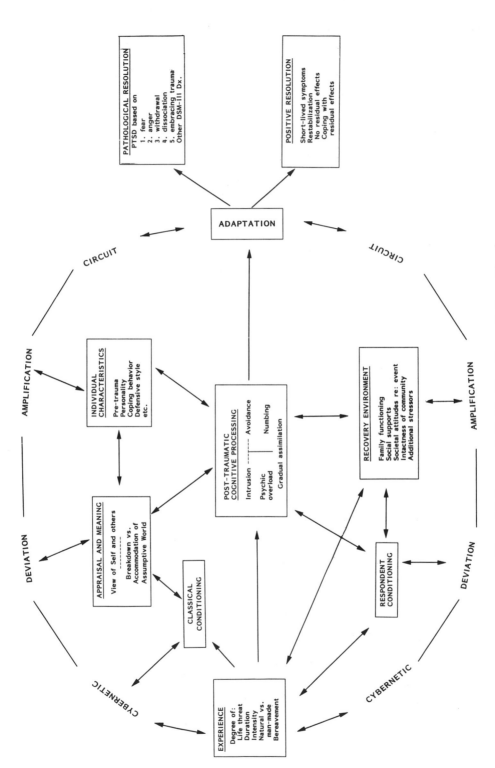

Figure 6.2. Ecosystemic Model of Post-Traumatic Stress Disorder

Janoff-Bulman (1985). There are three perspectives that are relevant. The first issue is the roles of the specific appraisals that the individual has made of the traumatic situation and the events that follow. Did the person believe that their life was in danger? Did the person find that the justice system was in fact just?

The second issue is closely related to the person's pre-trauma personality, coping behaviors, and defensive style. The important appraisals in this category revolve around how the person places the trauma, their behavior (cognitive, affective, and motoric), and the behavior of others in context with the rest of their life. Is the trauma just one more example of being victimized? Hendin et al. (1981) describe a case of a soldier who did not refuse to follow an order that violated standard procedure. The result was that two men were killed and the patient was wounded. The authors describe how the refusal to follow orders was part of a life-long pattern of resenting responsibility.

Certain attributions can be selectively utilized to maintain a specific coping response or defensive style. A woman who was injured on her job reacted with a great deal of anger to her employers. One of the central dynamics involved her assessments that: the employers had betrayed her; and, if she were to cry and feel her pain, that would mean that they had "beaten her." Therefore, she preferred to hang onto fantasies of revenge. This patient selectively preferred the intrusion of angry impulses in order to avoid her feelings of vulnerability.

An important variable that influences the severity of PTSD is how patients handle the fact that they have post-traumatic symptoms. Do they have characteristic attitudes that allow them to be in a needy position? Or, do they appraise the situation in such a manner that their previously positive views of themselves are further compromised? In other words, do they criticize themselves for not being strong enough? Does going to a psychologist lead them to believe they are crazy?

The third manner in which cognitive appraisal is important is on a macro-level. The degree to which the individual's assumptive world (Janoff-Bulman, 1985) or personal theory of reality (Epstein, 1989) is threatened will influence the cognitive processing of the trauma. The greater the breakdown of these basic beliefs the more likely the patient will be at the extremes of intrusion or numbing. The more flexible (or able to accommodate) the assumptive world, the more likely the traumatic experience can be assimilated. The degree of rigidity of defensive style, and the breadth of the repertoire of coping behaviors will influence vulnerability of the individual's basic beliefs.

Another possibilty is that the individual's personal theory of reality will accommodate too much. The result is that pathological changes in the personality structure will emerge (e.g., resolutions based on embracing the trauma). It is probable that when a person's basic beliefs are shattered they are more vulnerable to building new belief systems that have been contaminated by the traumatic event.

In Figure 6.2, different factors in the development of PTSD are surrounded by a cybernetic deviation amplification circuit (CDAC). This circuit can have a positive or negative direction effect. Furthermore, the degree of amplification can vary. While one can view the CDAC as a conduit for interaction between the different variables, it actually is more than a passive channel. Once the CDAC is established, "it" acts as if it had a mind of its own. It influences the other variables in a unidirectional manner with increasing amounts of amplitude. Furthermore, the stronger and more redundant the circuit, the more it will override any single change in other components.

Let us take two examples. In a negative outcome CDAC, a traumatized individual tends to appraise himself as weak and others as critical. He responds with avoidance. If someone tries to be understanding he sees them as pitying him. His response is to lash out at them in anger. The patient's wife is a relatively insecure woman, who needs approval. However, she really loves her husband. The sequence of events that sets the CDAC in motion is as follows:

1. The man has intrusive imagery.
2. He feels weak and believes others will criticize him for being weak.
3. He uses avoidance and withdraws.
4. His wife asks what is wrong.
5. He uses avoidance and anger, tells her to leave him alone.
6. His wife responds by feeling rejected and hurt. She starts to feel angry and ends up withdrawing also.

After a few cycles, the CDAC results in an amplification of her feelings of anger, and she become critical. This amplifies his avoidance and hostility and his sense of weakness, because now he can't stop her criticism, which was not even there before.

Even if, for a given moment, either one of them changes their behavior, the CDAC may prevent any systemic change. In fact, it can increase the amplification. For instance, one time the husband has a very bad nightmare. He decides for once he will tell his wife. She does not want to listen, because he pushed her away before he went to bed. She tells him to solve it himself. Now he "knows" she will be critical. Furthermore, he feels hurt and weak. He explodes and hits her. Now for the first time violence is part of the system.

A simple CDAC that results in a positive outcome can work as follows: A person is involved in a serious car crash. She has classically conditioned fear reactions. Her individual characteristics are such that she usually tries to overcome her fears. So she tries to drive in the car. Her fears overcome her. She leaves the car *before* her anxiety goes down. Fortunately, she is very close with a supportive friend, who happens to be a psychotherapist, who offers to drive with her. The first few times she feels a little better. She gains a little confidence. She becomes closer with her friend. One day, when they are out driving a car that looks exactly like the car that hit her gets a little too close. The woman becomes hysterical, and insists on leaving the car.

The friend not only knows that the flight response will hinder the problem but also feels that her professional esteem is on the line. She thinks, "After all, if you can't help your friend, what kind of a therapist are you." So now, there is no way that she is going to let her friend flee, *specifically because her friend is so upset.* She talks her friend down. The woman feels a sense of accomplishment for not having fled. Furthermore, she develops an alteration in her personal theory of reality. She knows that people really will help you when you need it most.

These examples of CDAC involve just a few variables. One can begin to appreciate how complicated a circuit can become when recognizing that there are multiple sources of intrapersonal and interpersonal variables that range from micro levels (e.g. learning principles,defensive operations or responses from different individuals) to macro levels (e.g. changes in assumptive beliefs or community responses).

Finally, we have expanded and differentiated the eventual adaptation. Following the discussion on the course of PTSD, pathological resolutions to trauma can take one of several forms. They can be based on the generalization of (1) fear; (2) withdrawal; (3) anger; (4) dissociation; and (5) embracing the trauma. Non-PTSD outcomes, such as major depression, can also occur.

Positive resolutions can take one of several forms. First, the patient can develop relatively mild symptoms that are short-lived. In this scenario, the patient has a post-traumatic reaction that is within a "normal" range. In other words, the person is appropriately upset by the trauma. In this type of positive outcome, the degree of disruption is minimal.

Second, after the development of PTSD, a healthy resolution involves restabilization. Individuals can return to their previous level of functioning. They may be free of residual symptoms. Or, they may have residual effects (e.g., occasional startle response, dreams, or periods of sadness) with which they cope effectively. The third outcome possibility involves genuine growth. In this event, as a result of working through the trauma, people reach a new level of maturity and functioning.

III

Assessment

7

The Assessment Process

INTRODUCTION

Before moving to the specific assessment process of PTSD, let us place this particular disorder in the context of evaluation in general. Before clinicians can go about making the detailed diagnostic assessment that will be discussed momentarily, they must be sensitized to the possibility that a patient *might* suffer from a trauma-related disorder.

For instance, some time ago when one of the authors was only beginning to focus his attention on PTSD, one of his patients described how she had identified with the Rod Steiger character in the movie *The Pawnbroker*. She had resonated with the experience of numbing of responsiveness. It so happens that this patient had been subjected to numerous reconstructive surgeries as a young child. All of a sudden it became perfectly clear that this woman was suffering from a chronic maladaptive resolution of PTSD that centered around denial and numbing. The author would never have picked this up had he not been sensitized to the issues of PTSD. Feeding this new information back to the patient and her family was helpful in the treatment process.

From our perspective, unless you know ahead of time that a probable differential diagnostic question is PTSD (e.g. someone referred for an accident evaluation, or rape evaluation) you need to be alert for clues of trauma to which clients allude. Or, you can ask several direct questions that will give you the desired information. (We will return to this later.)

There are different levels of assessment for any mental health problem; and PTSD is not an exception. We will discuss several different levels. These are:

1. screening for PTSD
2. formal DSM-III-R diagnosis
3. differential diagnosis
4. functional assessment of the individual
5. forensic evaluation

SCREENING

The central task in screening for PTSD involves discovering the existence of situations that are usually experienced as traumatic. The following questions should be answered, either as part of an open ended or a structured interview. If at this point there is sufficient evidence for further assessment, a more detailed diagnostic procedure is called for.

FORMAL DIAGNOSTIC PROCEDURE FOR DSM-III DIAGNOSIS

In this section we are focusing on the problem of establishing an effective protocol to accurately diagnose the presence of PTSD. In many cases and situations such a formal evaluation would not be necessary.

In order to achieve greater clarity, we have artificially separated the "formal diagnostic procedure for DSM-III-R classification" from the "functional assessment of the individual" (which will be discussed shortly). One style of assessment is to follow this procedure. In the preliminary evaluation, clinicians can follow the structured interview (and if necessary utilize formal psychological testing, and so on). In the following sessions, more idiosyncratic and functional information can be gathered. A second style of assessment would be to gather both types of information at the same time. As mentioned earlier, the context for the evaluation is likely to influence the type of information that will be given priority.

The assessment process described by T. Keane (personal communication, January 15, 1987) establishes a solid basis for the accurate diagnosis of PTSD. The process includes:

- a structured interview
- a formal mental status examination
- psychometric and psychodiagnostic testing (especially the utilization of instruments to differentiate PTSD from other disorders)
- multimethod behavioral assessment (behavioral, cognitive and psychophysiological measures)

Table 7.1. Questions for Screening of Trauma-Related Disorders

What is the most traumatic incident that has ever happened to you?	This question is the most general of the questions. Nevertheless, it presupposes that a person has had some trauma in his life, and asks the individual to search for the worst. To answer this question the person must compare and contrast any number of difficult situations that he has had. It is likely to yield a rich amount of associations.
What is the most traumatic incident that has ever happened to someone in your family?	A family member may come in for treatment, because the system has been destabilized by the trauma of someone else in the family.
Have you ever been a victim of a crime?	This question is self-evident.
Have you ever been in an accident serious enough so that you had to be medically examined?	Again this question is self-evident. Often people do not relate symptoms to events in their lives.
Have you ever served in the Armed Forces? If yes, In how much combat were you involved?	Another self-evident question. This question should also be asked of women. Many women have served in the armed forces.
Have you ever been as an adult or a child sexually assaulted?	Of course it is necessary to ask this type of question with sensitivity and tact. It most certainly should be asked of women, because there is perhaps as high as a one-in-four chance that an adult woman will have had at least one experience of sexual assault (Veronen & Kilpatrick,1983). It also would not be a bad idea to ask this of men. The amount of sexual abuse of boys is certainly underreported.
At any point during this (these) experience(s) did you think you were in danger of serious personal harm or losing your life?	In their study of the effects of crime on women, Kilpatrick et al. (in press) found that the one factor that most correlated with PTSD was the cognitive appraisal that the victim was in danger of serious personal injury or loss of life. In fact, if forced to ask just one question, Kilpatrick (personal communication, Feb 26, 1988) would ask whether the individual ever felt that he was in jeopardy of serious personal harm or loss of life.

Although this model is derived from work with combat veterans, it is generalizable to other PTSD patient populations, especially those with chronic or delayed sub-types.

STRUCTURED INTERVIEW

The first aspect of this assessment involves a structured interview. With respect to patient information, the following detailed information should be collected:

- demographic information
- medical history
- disability status
- employment history
- social history
- educational history

Figley (1985) suggests various specific data be collected with respect to PTSD patients. Although the format Figley (1985) suggests is again oriented toward Vietnam veterans, it is presented here more generally so that it might be adapted to other patient populations with PTSD. The interview is based directly on the primary and secondary features of PTSD noted in Chapters 1 and 2. In essence, the examiner asks detailed questions about each aspect of PTSD symptomatology, specifying nature, content, frequency, intensity, duration, vicissitudes, and brief descriptions of all symptoms. The format suggested contains specific questions related to:

- the nature and degree of exposure to traumatic experience
- specific trauma central to PTSD symptomatology
- PTSD symptoms
  - intrusive thoughts, feelings, images, memories
  - numbing of responsiveness
  - avoidance responses
- associated features
  - depression
  - anxiety
  - aggression
  - substance abuse
- pre-morbid adjustment
  - school performance
  - pre-morbid social life
  - pre-morbid family life
  - family history of mental illness

The data gleaned from the structured interview form the basis of the assessment and diagnostic procedure. The greater the awareness of the symptoms, subtypes, and course of PTSD, the greater the examiner's ability to accurately and validly assess the disorder. This basic structure can be adapted for each of the various types of traumatic stressor and specific responses; it may also be expanded to include more secondary features or more detailed information.

FORMAL MENTAL STATUS EXAMINATION

The formal mental status examination utilized in the assessment procedures with patients manifesting PTSD is standard, including questions related to: orientation, sensory experiences, motor functions, emotions and mood, delusional behavior, mathematical skills, proverbs, judgment, memory (auditory, visual), visual-spatial skills.

The information collected during the mental status examination often provides important data pertaining to the cognitive functioning of the patient.

PSYCHOMETRIC AND PSYCHODIAGNOSTIC TESTING

To further diagnostic certainty, patients suspected of manifesting PTSD may be administered various psychological tests. Traditional batteries of tests can provide information overlooked or missed during the structured interview and mental status examination. More diagnostically reliable data are collected from MMPI records since PTSD patients often manifest a characteristic pattern.

Traditional Batteries

Little has been written about the performance of patients with PTSD on standard intellectual and projective tests. Bailey (1985) notes that patients with PTSD often show anxiety interference on the digit span subtest of the WAIS-R. More has been written about the performance of patients with PTSD on the Rorschach.

Van der Kolk and Ducey (1984) note that the subjects tested in their study, Vietnam veterans with PTSD, fell into two basic categories of experience type, extratensive and coarcted. Markedly extratensive protocols were characterized by:

• extensive, unstructured use of color

- high number of CF responses (color-form)[9]
- virtual absence of M responses (human movement)[10]
- extensive blood and anatomy content
- uncensored and uncontrolled references to traumatic Vietnam experiences
- high numbers of M responses (inanimate movement responses)
- an absence of well integrated responses

Despite the above, psychosis was not indicated in these patients. Characteristics of coarcted protocols included:

- very few responses
- no color responses
- little/no M responses (human movement responses)

Van der Kolk and Ducey (1984) described these two types of styles as "mirror images" of each other. Their findings confirm behavioral observations of PTSD regarding denial-numbing and intrusive phases. They are summarized as follows with reference to their Vietnam veteran subjects:

- Ambiguous/affectively charged stimuli promote the recurrence of traumatic stress.
- People with PTSD cannot modulate affective experience.
- If patients respond to affective experience they do so with an intensity appropriate to the traumatic situation (i.e.,intrusive feelings; lack of affect tolerance).
- Alternatively, patients do not respond to affective stimuli at all (i.e., psychic numbing).
- The capacity to symbolize, fantasize, or sublimate is markedly diminished.
- The psychological mechanisms that allow people to cope with the narcissistic injuries of life are missing.

Bailey (1985) adds that the Rorschach responses of Vietnam veteran patients with PTSD often contain emotionally charged war-related perceptions. Van der Kolk and Ducey (1984) note that with patients characterized by emotional constriction, the use of the Rorschach may indicate the presence of PTSD which would have been missed otherwise.

MMPI

Studies which have employed the MMPI to assess the adjustment of patients with PTSD have consistently shown elevated scores on a number of clinical scales (Penk et al., 1981; Fairbank, Keane & Malloy, 1983).

However, the subject samples in these studies tended to be small, or the subjects characterized by specific clinical features (e.g., alcoholism).

The following scales are relevant for PTSD. The F-scale was originally designed to detect deviant or atypical thinking. High scores on the scale can be interpreted in several ways: (1) attempts to fake-bad (e.g. malingering, or exaggerating symptoms to ask for help); (2) random responding; (3) may manifest severely neurotic or psychotic thinking.

The K-Scale measures attempts to present oneself in a favorable light. Low scores may indicate a person is either exaggerating problems as a plea for help, trying to fake bad, or is self-critical, suspicious, ineffective with dealing with problems of daily life.

Scale 2 or D measures symptomatic depression. Scale 8 or Sc is termed the schizophrenia scale. It measures psychotic symptoms such as hallucinations. However, it also measures social alienation, fears, difficulties with impulse control, and concentration (Graham, 1977).

In Keane, Malloy, and Fairbank's (1984) study of 100 Vietnam veterans with PTSD and 100 psychiatric controls, a consistent MMPI-8-2 pattern was noted in the PTSD group. The F clinical scale was also consistently, and significantly, elevated. In addition, significantly higher scores were noted on all clinical scales except Mf, and significantly lower scores on K. The decision rule developed included cutoff scores at:

- F = 66T
- Sc (8) = 79T
- D (2) = 78T

Subjects with all three scores above the cutoff levels were classified as having PTSD. This decision rule led to the correct identification of approximately 75% of the patients with PTSD. Keane, Malloy, and Fairbank (1984) note that clinicians wishing for greater accuracy can use higher cutoff scores on the F, D (2), and Sc (8) clinical scales. The result, though, is increased false negative rates.

Hyer et al. (1986) also found that inpatient veterans with PTSD also had elevated 8-2 patterns on their MMPI. The respective mean T-scores were 101.6 and 100.6. Not only were these scores statistically higher than for inpatient combat and noncombat veterans, they were significantly different at a clinical level. The mean T-scores for the non-PTSD groups on the 8 and 2 scales were approximately 25 and 20 points lower.

PTSD subscale of the MMPI. Keane, Malloy, and Fairbank (1984) also developed a special subscale for combat-related PTSD. The hit rate of this scale was over 80%. They note that the items included on the scale tended to relate directly to the major PTSD criteria in the DSM-III-R. In sum, Keane, Malloy, and Fairbank (1984) note that the MMPI could reliably discriminate the PTSD group from veterans with affective disorders, anxiety disorders, personality disorders, and psychotic disorders. Hyer et al. (1986) also found that the MMPI-PTSD subscale could accurately differentiate inpatient veteran with PTSD from other inpatient combat and non-combat veterans without PTSD. However, the hit rate was somewhat lower 69%.

Multimethod Behavioral Assessment

The multimethod behavioral assessment procedure developed by Malloy, Fairbank, and Keane (1983) includes:

- behavioral measures
- cognitive measures
- psychophysiological measures

This tripartite assessment was used to diagnose combat-related PTSD in Vietnam veterans. This type of assessment is mostly suited for specialized centers and/or research purposes. The tripartite assessment procedure involves exposing Vietnam veterans to slides of war-related activities and neutral scenes (recorded on videotape). Patients are permitted to terminate exposure to the trauma-evoking stimuli (the behavioral measure). Subjectively reported anxiety ratings are collected for both war-related and neutral slides using the Subjective Units of Distress Scale (SUDS) (the cognitive measure). Finally, the patient's heart rate and skin resistance level are monitored (the psychophysiological measure).

Although this tripartite assessment procedure requires specialized equipment, it provides a wealth of valuable data for examiners. Both the behavioral measures (escape from traumatic stimulus) and the behavioral measures (heart rate and skin resistance) are extremely important. Malloy et al. (1983) were able correctly to discriminate subjects with PTSD from controls with 90% accuracy with the behavioral criteria of terminating the trauma-evoking stimuli before they were over. Controls were always able to watch the traumatic scenes. Using just physiological measures, an 80% hit rate was achieved. The usefulness of psychophysiological measures have been supported by others (Blanchard et al., 1982; Kolb & Multipassi, 1982).

Paper and Pencil Inventories

There have been many different inventories and assessment tools that have been used to evaluate PTSD. However, several instruments tend to be used more often than others. Furthermore, they are relatively brief. They also are particularly relevant to PTSD. The Impact of Events Scale (IES) (Horowitz, 1986) directly measures the degree of intrusion and avoidance that patients experience. There are both self-report and clinician-report versions.

The Reaction Index (RI) is a self-report inventory based on the diagnostic criteria for PTSD in DSM-III (Frederick, 1985, 1987). It consists of 20 questions that are answered on a five-point scale, ranging from none of the time to most of the time. Items include questions about intrusive experience, fears and tension, and avoidance and numbing. It was standardized using 300 subjects from 5 groups: POW's, physical assault victims, disaster victims, hostages and rape victims. In one study (Frederick, 1987) using 50 cases, 10 from each group, the scores of the subjects correlated 0.87 with the MMPI-PTSD scale (Keane, Malloy, & Fairbank, 1984). This finding is particularly interesting, because the Keane study was assessing Vietnam veterans, whereas the Frederick study had five different types of victims. One potential conclusion is that from a symptomatic picture across different groups may not be that different. A score of 25 and above was the cutoff for the RI for inclusion in the PTSD group. A score of 40 and above is indicative of a severe case with a 98% probability of PTSD. Scores of 35 or higher indicate a 87% probability of PTSD.

The Veronen-Kilpatrick modified Fear Survey (Veronen & Kilpatrick, 1980) has been used most often in clinical research involving rape. The Beck Depression Inventory has also been used frequently. While not addressing PTSD directly, it is a quick instrument that allows the clinician to readily document and track the degree of depression a patient is experiencing.

DIFFERENTIAL DIAGNOSIS

PTSD must often be differentiated from other DSM-III-R diagnostic categories. Common diagnostic differentials include:

- anxiety disorders
- depressive disorders
- adjustment disorders
- antisocial personality disorders
- schizophrenia
- factitous PTSD
- malingering

Each of these differential diagnoses will be discussed in more detail.

Anxiety Disorders

The central difference between PTSD and the other anxiety disorders is the presence of a specified trauma (which is not a criterion for generalized anxiety disorder or panic disorder) and the specificity of the types of symptoms. DSM-III advises that if the anxiety is severe enough, an anxiety disorder can also be diagnosed. However, we feel this does not make much sense, because it does not add any new information. Nor does it provide option for different types of treatment. The possible exception, may be panic disorder, which may suggest the use of medication to block the panic. It must be discerned whether agoraphobic symptoms are result of trauma, as in rape. If they are then PTSD should be the primary diagnosis.

Depressive Disorders

Depression routinely coexists with PTSD (Sierles et al., 1986). DSM-III-R notes that depressive disorders that coexist with PTSD should be diagnosed. The most germane disorder for discernment is major depression. The most relevant signs that are likely to stand out from PTSD symptomatology are the vegetative signs of depression (e.g., terminal insomnia,[11] changes in appetite, fatigue, loss of pleasure in usually pleasurable activities), thoughts of death or suicide, positive family history for depression. The most important reason for making this additional diagnosis would be the proper use of antidepressive medication.

Adjustment Disorders

Clinically, this differential diagnosis may be one of the most difficult. There are two dimensions on which these diagnoses differ: degree of stressor and types of symptomatology. It will actually be clearer if we take the second dimension first. Regardless of the degree of the stressor, the diagnosis of PTSD can *only* be given if the person exhibits the *characteristic* symptoms of PTSD. These include: reexperiencing the trauma, avoidance of stimuli associated with the trauma, or psychic numbing, and increased arousal (not present before the trauma). If the person is simply not functioning as well, if he or she is just somewhat depressed or anxious or does not concentrate or work as well, then the diagnosis of adjustment disorder is more reasonable.

The first dimension is the level of the stressor. For an adjustment disorder the stressor merely needs to be identifiable. For PTSD the criterion for the stressor is that it be outside of the range of usual human experience and would be markedly distressing to almost anyone. The DSM-III-R states that in adjustment disorder the stressor is usually less severe.

At the extremes of the continuum of stressors, it is clear which criteria are out of the range of normal human experience (e.g., torture, rape, collapse of a building, and so on) and which criteria are within the normal range of experience (e.g., family problems, divorce, difficulty with business). However, there are areas that are difficult to discern, and, in fact, are mentioned under both adjustment disorder and PTSD in the DSM-III-R. The main area of confusion is illness and death of a loved one. While there is virtually no empirical evidence at the present time, we would like to present some guidelines for differentiating these stressors, with a strong caveat that they are only guidelines, and are open to revision.

To the extent that the loss or illness is part of normal developmental processes (i.e., aging) the more likely criterion A for PTSD is *not* being met. In fact, the DSM-III-R lists simple bereavement as an experience that is within the range of normal experience. The more the illness or loss is unsynchronized with expected development (e.g., a young child dying) the more likely criterion A for PTSD *is* being met.

The more the illness is a result of human negligence, the more likely criterion A for PTSD is being fulfilled. Let us look at an unusual and difficult example that will raise an important issue. Worker A develops some sort of illness that is associated with his work, but only rarely. Worker A had been duly informed of the possibility of risk, and was promptly attended to by the employers in a responsible manner. On the other hand, worker B who gets sick as a function of their job, was never informed of this risk. In fact, worker B was assured that the job was *absolutely* safe, even though the employer knew otherwise. A conflictual relationship develops between the employers and worker B. The level of stress in worker B's case is more likely to meet criterion A for PTSD, because worker B's expectation was that the environment was safe. Additionally, there is the added burden of the realizing that the world is unjust.

In the actual case, worker B also met the remaining criteria for PTSD. The issue we are presenting here is that events need to given meaning before they are experienced as stressful or not. As we have already described, PTSD appears to occur because of the breakdown in the individual's assumptive world (Janoff-Bulman, 1985; Epstein, 1989). In the case just described, worker B had, in fact, been highly trusting of her employers. When it became clear that they had lied about the hazardousness of the materials with which she worked, her assumptions about the trustworthiness of people were shattered. Furthermore, there was significant secondary victimization (additional stress beyond the initial trauma), by the adversarial positions that developed (see p. 126 for further discusssion). In the case of worker A, there was less of a chance of basic assumptions becoming fragmented.

Let us look at this problem from a different angle. The DSM-III-R states that the trauma must be outside the range of usual experience. What about people whose line of work often places them in situations outside the realm of usual experience. Two obvious examples include fireman and policeman. Being caught in the middle of an inferno would surely meet criteria A for most of us. If an experienced fireman is overcome by smoke in a blaze, would that be outside of the realm of usual experience for a fireman? The answer is not all that clear. One might raise the same question about policemen and being involved in a gunfight. We are not going to resolve the question here. However, we do feel it is worth raising.

Antisocial Personality Disorder

The differentiation of PTSD from antisocial personality disorders is difficult (Walker, 1981a). The confusion between the two disorders (at least in Vietnam veterans) is often increased by the presence of:

- hostile attitudes
- difficulties with authority
- a history of substance abuse
- frequent difficulties with the law
- disrupted object relations
- sexual difficulties
- failure to honor financial obligations
- reckless behavior
- impulsivity

Some argue that antisocial personality disorder may also be routinely expected to coexist with PTSD (Sierles et al., 1986). Bailey (1985) suggests two procedures to facilitate the differential with Vietnam veterans. The first involves a thorough social history inquiry. Characteristics of veterans with an antisocial personality disorder include:

- poor premilitary history (e.g., truancy, institutionalization)
- forced into service
- chose service to escape an unpleasant circumstance
- no history of combat
- with history of combat, vague recollections of the experience
- onset of symptoms throughout premilitary and military periods

In contrast, characteristics of veterans with PTSD include:

- good premilitary history (e.g., good school record, involvement)
- joined service for patriotic reasons
- joined service through draft
- history of combat
- with history of combat, specific recollections of combat experiences
- onset of symptoms in postmilitary period

Walker (1981) also stresses the need to contrast the adolescent history of the veteran (especially, the years prior to age 15) with current personality features (especially, those manifested after the age of 18 and during the past 5 years).

Differences also exist in current symptomatology. Antisocial personality-disordered veterans tend to be characterized by:

- a lack of guilt
- emphasis on changing environment
- strong feelings expressed for manipulative reasons
- severity of war trauma easily presented

In contrast, the characteristics of veterans with PTSD include:

- guilt/survivor guilt
- an emphasis on changing self
- emotional numbing
- combat experiences presented with difficulty and only after trust established

Goodwin (1980) and Walker (1981) have made similar observations regarding the current clinical presentation of PTSD patients and antisocial personality-disordered patients.

Finally, Bailey (1985) indicates differences between veterans with antisocial personality disorders and PTSD on psychodiagnostic testing. The antisocial personality disorder group manifested:

- MMPI: pathological elevations on subscales 4, 8, 2
- projectives: few fabulized answers
- projectives: manipulative story themes
- WAIS-R: no anxiety inference on digit span

In contrast, PTSD veterans manifested (Bailey, 1985; Keane et al., 1984):

- MMPI: an F, 2, 8 pattern (with elevations on all clinical scales except 5)
- projective tests: strong fabulized war-related responses
- WAIS-R: anxiety inference on digit span

Many of the same diagnostic procedures employed for the differential between PTSD and antisocial personality disorder may be employed to differentiate PTSD from borderline personality disorder. Again, however, the frequent similarity in presentation often makes differentiation difficult.

Schizophrenia

DeFazio (1978) and Domash and Sparr (1982) note that PTSD may be confused with forms of schizophrenia (e.g., paranoid schizophrenia). They note that the initial presenting picture between schizophrenia and severe PTSD may be strikingly similar, and lead to the implementation of innapropriate treatment plans. Van Putten and Emory (1973) have noted three characteristics inherent in stress response syndromes which give them a superficial resemblance to schizophrenic processes:

- contraction of ego functioning resembling schizophrenic deterioration (e.g., inability to handle the activities of daily living and subsequent withdrawal
- phobic elaboration of events which characterize the world as hostile and persecutory often resembles psychotic persecutory delusions
- explosive rage reactions in altered states is sometimes confused with "psychomotor epilepsy"

Clearly this is particularly relevant to those who survived the death camps, the bombings of Hiroshima and Nagasaki, and high levels of combat in the Vietnam war with witnessing of/participation in atrocities. Although Domash and Sparr (1982) do not delineate procedures for differentiating the two disorders, a thorough social history may provide the necessary data for so doing. Another important factor is the continuity of trauma-related concerns into the current clinical picture in cases of PTSD.

Factitious PTSD and Malingering

In both malingering and factitious disorders patients produce the symptoms voluntarily. The central difference is that with factitious disorders the only purpose for producing the disorder appears to be to take the "patient role." It is almost always associated with severe personality disorder (APA, 1987). Malingering patients have an obvious goal that involves secondary gain. These goals include: financial remuneration, evasion of criminal prosecution, or the procurement of drugs (APA, 1987).

The issue of whether or not a person is malingering or whether the diagnosis of PTSD is "accurate" is most often a concern about money. The issue comes up in regard to veterans disability payments and legal cases that involve monetary damages.

Sparr and Pankratz (1983) report on the difficulties inherent in differentiating PTSD from factitious PTSD. They note that since the delineation of PTSD as a separate diagnostic category, various attempts have been made by patients to fabricate the disorder at Veterans Administration facilities. Within the sample of subjects discussed, all patients blatantly misrepresented facts.

Faking combat PTSD can be *best* discerned by a careful history that includes that actual procurement of records, in particular the national prisoner of war registry and discharge papers (form DD214) (Sparr & Pankratz, 1983; Pary, Tobias, & Lippman, 1987).

It has been suggested that if patients have T-scores above 88 on the F-scale it indicates they are exaggerating symptoms and the diagnosis of PTSD is suspect (Fairbank, McCaffrey & Keane, 1985; Pary et al., 1987). However, Hyer et al. (1987) found that 50% of veterans independently diagnosed with PTSD scored in the exaggerated range.

Kean, Malloy and Fairbank (1984) developed a 49-item MMPI-PTSD scale. Using a cutoff score of 30, they were able to correctly classify 82% of the patients tested. However, in a cross-validation study, Hyer et al. (1986) only had a hit rate of 69%. It is common that the validity of a test will shrink as it is cross-validated. This raises the question of just how much more inaccurate will these measures be when they are being used to differentiate "fakers" from "real" cases.

Hyer et al. (1987) found equivocal results in their study of MMPI overreporting by Vietnam Veterans. They advocated caution when using the MMPI-PTSD sub scale because they found that 50% of PTSD veterans had F-scales[12] in the exaggerated range (T-score of 88 or greater). However, they also found that PTSD veterans when compared to noncombat and non-PTSD veterans did not respond differentially to obvious and neutral (more subtle) items on the scale. This finding implied that PTSD veterans simply endorse many items on the F-scale, but are not necessarily faking bad. Therefore, at least in combat cases, symptom overreporting is not necessarily a robust tool for discerning factitious PTSD.

The conclusions that must be reached at this point are that it is difficult to discern factitious from real PTSD. It is best to use multiple methods and make a clinical judgment based on the pattern that evolves from the various different sources of information.

The discussion of differentiating faking from bona fide PTSD needs to be placed in its proper context. This becomes especially clear in regard to the problem with veterans faking disability. The amount of money at stake is considerable. A veteran on full disability payments receives approximately $1500 a month tax free. Over 25 years this amounts to just under half a million dollars per veteran. Therefore, it is understandable that the Veterans Administration would want to ferret out malingerers. However, experienced nurses will also report the interesting phenomenon of patients who have not been to the hospital in years suddenly becoming ill as their reevaluation comes up. The system is set up so that, once hospitalized, a veteran's benefits are automatically raised to 100% disability. From a behavioral science point of view, the wrong contingencies of reinforcement are being used. The conclusion that one must suspect is, that psychologists and psychiatrists are being asked to make differentiations to compensate for the inefficiencies of a bureaucratic system.

The controversy becomes even more interesting if we refer to the study of Zusman and Simon (1983). They looked at the conflicting assessments of victims of the Buffalo Creek disaster (the plaintiffs) by clinicians for the plaintiffs and the defense. All of the clinicians were reputable and had little reason to distort their findings. The plaintiffs were evaluated in two groups. The first group were evaluated three and a half years after the flood (plaintiffs Team A). The second group of people were evaluated 18 months later (plaintiffs Team B). All of the plaintiffs were evaluated by the defense two months later. The findings included:

1. There was a continuum of reported flood-related symptomatology, with plaintiffs Team A finding the most, the defendant teams finding the least, and plaintiffs Team B in between.
2. With respect to the evaluation of recovery, there was a significant difference between the plaintiffs Teams assessment (65.5 and 76.9% no recovery, and 34.5 and 23.1% partial recovery) versus the defendants assessment (19% no recovery, 35.7% partial recovery, 21% complete recovery, 23.8% never ill).

Zusman and Simon (1983) suggested that there were three reasons that these differences occur. First, plaintiffs team A, unlike all the other teams, conducted their interviews in the home in conjoint interviews. The conjoint interview was described as the "most effective" method for "uncovering psychologically relevant material because West Virginia mining area culture 'encourages reticence about personal feelings...especially to outsiders'" (p 1303).

Given the strength of these findings, Zusman and Simon were surprised that their influence was not found throughout the analysis. Second, the orientation of the psychiatrists of the plaintiffs was analytic, whereas the defendants' psychiatrists were eclectic. Third, the evidence strongly suggested partisanship. It was felt that while the examiners may have started out neutral, they did not remain that way. Zusman and Simon (1983) termed this forensic identification. They felt this was an artifact of the adversarial system.

The issue of examiner bias is important on a number of levels. One dimension is that there are demand characteristics (Orne, 1969) placed on clinicians in a court case that may subtly and unconsciously influence data selection and interpretive relevance. A second dimension is that the different examiners from the different sides will exert different demand characteristics on the patients. It is not unlikely then that there will be in actuality different data. A third perspective is that outside the forensic arena the diagnostic emphasis will not be on whether or not the person is faking. For instance, much more attention is likely to be placed on evaluating the person's strengths and resources or their particular needs for therapy. (A discussion on forensic evaluations of PTSD appears on page 129)

Finally, having looked at the issue of discerning sham versus real PTSD, it needs to be reiterated that at this time the central problem with the diagnosis of PTSD is that it is underdiagnosed. It is not uncommon for patients finally to come for treatment for one reason or another. And, they do not report that they had been in Vietnam, or had been sexually abused or raped, or traumatized in one fashion or another. It may be that they are consciously concealing the trauma, dissociating or repressing its occurrence, or do not think it is relevant to their "current" problem.

FUNCTIONAL EVALUATION OF THE INDIVIDUAL

The identification of a patient as suffering from PTSD is not the end of the evaluation. In fact, it is just the beginning. The next goal is a functional evaluation of the individual for treatment planning. We will follow the parameters outlined by Scurfield (1985)[13] in performing such an evaluation.

Pre-Trauma History

A pre-trauma history involves two types of goals . The first is to establish the person's pre-morbid functioning. This information will be useful for two reason. One reason is to determine if a personality disorder is also evident. The second reason is to know what the person's baseline of functioning has been. If the therapy is relatively brief the goal will be to return the person to their pre-morbid level of adjustment (Horowitz, 1986). The second goal for inquiry into pre-trauma history is to discover the common themes of the person's conflicts or life struggles. While the PTSD may be largely due to a current stressor, the expression of the symptoms and their elaborations in the patient's life will be significantly influenced by the patient's characteristic modes of coping and attribution (Horowitz, 1986).

Immediate Pre-Trauma Psychosocial Context

Scurfield (1985) rightly points out the importance of assessing the trauma victim's psychosocial context at the time of the trauma. What was the person's age, level of development? We would add: What was the level of development of the person's family system? What were the developmental hurdles with which the person was dealing or about to face (e.g., leaving home, getting married, and so on)?

The Event and the Immediate Coping Responses

There are several factors that must be assessed.

"Objective" Factors. The objective factors consist of the frequency, duration, intensity and nature of the trauma. Areas of inquiry include:

- Was it a single or multiple trauma?
- Were the traumas clearly delineated incidents? or
- Was the trauma a culmination of a number of experiences?
- Was the trauma human induced or an act of nature? (Scurfield, 1985)
- Did it occur to only one individual or a group?

Active/Passive Role. The degree of passivity versus activity can have a powerful influence on the meaning of the trauma and the development of PTSD (Ayalon, 1983; Figley, 1985). Did the patient act as a helpless victim? Was he or she active in any way to alter the situation? Were there any options for acting differently? How did/does the patient perceive the meaning and outcome of his or her actions?

Idiosyncratic Meaning of the Trauma. In this area of inquiry clinicians are assessing the specific idiosyncratic meanings of the trauma situation. For example, Horowitz (1986) describes a man who was in an accident after picking up a woman hitchhiker. She died in the crash. One of the possible idiosyncratic meanings was that he was having sexual fantasies about the woman.

Post-Trauma Psychosocial Context

The recovery environment is an important aspect in the overall readjustment of individuals with PTSD (Green et al., 1985; Scurfield, 1985). Relevant areas include the responses of the family (Figley, 1988), the community (Ayalon, 1983), social agency responses (Kilpatrick et al., 1989; Quarenteli, 1985).

Family Responses. Figley (1988) has described four functions that the family can provide in the healing of PTSD. Actually, he has elaborated the healing side of four variables that influence the course of PTSD. We will add the negative side of the continuum. Part of an evaluation is to determine where the family is on the different dimensions.

Healing	*Pathology*
1. Detecting traumatic stress symptoms	Denying/discounting existence or importance of stress symptoms
2. Confronting the trauma	Denying/discounting the need to deal with the trauma
3. Urging recapitulation of the catastrophe	Reinforcing avoidance and numbing
4. Facilitating resolution of conflicts	Actively avoids conflict resolution or poor skills lead to conflict escalation

Another dimension that is relevant is the degree to which the family has been "infected" by the trauma (Figley, 1988) versus the degree to which the traumatized person has been supported by the family. In other words, to what extent has the family system been structurally reorganized around the trauma so that the functioning of the family members becomes impaired. For example, has the result of the nightmares of a traumatized child been that mother and father can no longer function as husband and wife (e.g. not have sex)? Or, have the parents been able to help the child resolve the nightmares?

Responses from Social Agencies. Most individuals who have been traumatized or victimized come in contact with some agency of society, such as the Veterans Administration, the criminal/legal system, insurance companies, doctors and social agencies. Secondary victimization is a problem that occurs. Clinicians need to know the quality of the experience that patients had when dealing with these agencies. Were they treated with respect? Were they satisfied with their treatment? Were they ridiculed or told to "knock it off, and get on with life"? In secondary victimization, the individual is victimized once by the original stressor, then a second time by the responses of others.

Community Responses. It can be important to know the overall cultural and community expectations in which PTSD patients live. What is the community reaction to the trauma in question? What is the community expectation of the appropriate responses and roles of themselves and the victim? To what extent has the community accepted or rejected the patient?

Assessment of Attribution of Meaning

The attributions of meaning that the PTSD patient has are important variables to understand for the therapeutic process. Following Epstein (1988) and Janoff-Bulman (1985), it is important to discover the idiosyncratic elaborations of the pre-morbid basic assumptions, and then the extent to which the trauma has altered them. Is the person still confused and dazed? Or, are there new personal outlooks in place? What are the new views about the self and the world? Has the person made a resolution around a pathological assumption (e.g., the world is dangerous and I am weak).

It is also important to evaluate the attributions regarding responsibility for the trauma. What are the attributions with respect to the meaning of the trauma? A most important question is, what does the trauma mean in terms of the victims' plans for the rest of their life (Veronen & Kilpatrick, 1983)? Is the person focused on the unfairness of past or on the possibilities of the future?

Assessing Strengths and Resources

It is important also to evaluate patients' strengths and resources from a number of perspectives. In some instances significant positive outcomes can have occurred as a result of trauma (Scurfield, 1985; Veronen & Kilpatrick, 1983). These can include: comradeship, an increased sense of integrity, development of strong convictions and a healthy questioning or reaffirmation of one's values (Scurfield, 1985). A point of trauma can also be viewed as a choice point in life, where new directions can be taken (Veronen & Kilpatrick, 1983).

Clinicians can also make the mistake of focusing too much on problem states, while forgetting about solution or health states (de Shazer, 1985). Professionals can underestimate the amount of positive emotion that traumatized individuals normally experience. (Wortman & Silver, 1987). In looking for resources, relevant questions include asking: When does the person feel better, even if it is the exception and not the rule (de Shazer, 1985)? What thoughts and behaviors have they at those times? What coping strategies have been tried that were even partially successful? What other difficult situations has the person overcome in the past? What resources were used at that time?

Bandura (1977, 1982) describes two forms of efficacy. The first, outcome efficacy, is defined as the belief that there is a response to the stressor that will alleviate the problem. The second, efficacy expectation, is defined as the belief that the individual can successfully perform the needed response.

In assessing the resources of the PTSD patient, the clinician needs to evaluate the degree to which:

1. The patient believes a response exists that will alleviate their suffering (outcome efficacy).
2. The patient believes it is within his power to perform the response (efficacy expectation).

If outcome efficacy is low, the therapeutic enterprise may be more focused on skill development. If efficacy expectation is low, the therapeutic effort may be more focused on motivation or attitudinal change.

ASSESSMENT OF PTSD IN FORENSIC SITUATIONS: ETHICAL GUIDELINES AND METHODOLOGIES[14]

Ethical Issues Working for the Defense

Generally the defendant in a legal case is an insurance company or government. Certainly, the more famous cases involve the state or federal government using expert witnesses in criminal court. However, most cases involve a plaintiff suing for damages and/or payment of medical and psychological services on the basis of some type of post-traumatic stress disorder. The defendant (usually an insurance company) is trying to limit the amount of money paid to the plaintiff.

Motives for limitations or nonpayment of claims or damages vary. Former insurance adjusters and adjuster supervisors report that one large motive is simply mercenary. The insurer makes more money if they pay less money in claims. The ends justify the means in these cases. There is no regard for ethical or legal responsibilities. A second motive is that the insurer genuinely believes that the case is fraudulent. A third motive is that the insurer recognizes that the plaintiff may have some claim to damages, but not to the extent that he is claiming. For one of these reasons, insurers or their lawyers hire clinicians to make their own examinations.

Clearly, the client with the latter two motives will present fewer ethical dilemmas for the psychologist than a client with the first type of motive. Discussions with lawyers or former adjusters for insurance companies reveal that there are informal lists of psychologists and psychiatrists who are "hired guns." The "hired gun" will put in his or her report what the client desires, regardless of its veracity. Some clients will prefer an honest report. The client with the mercenary mentality is likely to use a "hired gun."

The job of the clinician when working for the insurer is to provide an *independent* exam. Unfortunately, all too often examiners are far from independent. There are subtle and not so subtle forms of pressure brought to bear. We have already discussed the issue of forensic identification. Another problem is that the clinician may be interested in having more than one referral from a particular lawyer or insurance company. The client then has potential leverage over the clinician. In many instances this is communicated subtly or indirectly. In other cases it is made blatantly clear. Psychologists are not immune to the pressure of social influence. Cognitive dissonance also influences professionals. Therefore, if you want to remain clearly within ethical boundaries, we recommend that you associate only with ethical clients. There is much to be said for the adversarial roles of the courts. Clinicians should not be afraid of being involved in a "good" fight. The ethical question is whether or not it is a "fair" fight.

Ethical Issues Working for the Plaintiff

It would be naive to think that clinicians working for plaintiffs are not under economic pressure to perform for their client. There are lists of "hired guns" for plaintiffs. There are lawyers who will exert pressure through offering or withholding further resources. There is the additional pressure of sometimes not getting paid (by the insurance carrier) for an evaluation if the finding is that there is *not* evidence for PTSD. Everything that we have recommended in regard to defense work regarding these issues equally applies to plaintiff work.

In many respects, working for the plaintiff often *feels* ethically easier than working for the defense. After all, it is one client against the "big, bad" insurance company.

Furthermore, if the client loses they may not be able to afford treatment. Most psychologists are emotionally and professionally in support of clients getting treatment. In addition, many psychologist just do not think in adversarial terms. They also do not think that people would be deliberately faking symptoms. Even if the symptoms were exaggerated due to secondary gain, the process is viewed as nonvolitional.

An Appropriate Mind-Set for Forensic Evaluations

The most appropriate frame of reference of the psychologist conducting a forensic evaluation is that of an experimenter who starts off accepting the null hypothesis. The null hypothesis in this situation is that the patient is normal. The examiner then gathers the data. The two central questions are: Is there significant deviation from the norm? Can the deviations found be linked to the trauma?

As we have already said, there are differential pressures on the defense and plaintiff examiners. It would be naive to think that there is one truth. It would also be naive to think that examiner bias can be totally eliminated. Therefore, we suggest that the bias be recognized in the same manner as it is in experimental settings, namely the alpha level.[15]

In other words, examiners for the plaintiff will tend to be more lenient in the degree of certainty needed to reject the null hypothesis (probably in the range equivalent to 0.05 to 0.01). Examiners for the defense will tend to use stricter criteria for rejecting the null hypothesis (on the order of 0.001). Obviously, we are using these numbers in a metaphoric sense. Nevertheless, they do reflect the range of variance that is appropriate and ethical. For instance, to be using criteria that are either so strict that they would be equivalent to an alpha level of 0.0001, or so lenient so that they would be equivalent to an alpha level of 0.10, would hardly meet the criteria normally set for scientific purposes.

The Forensic Evaluation of PTSD

Several different perspectives on evaluating PTSD have already been presented. These forms of assessment (e.g., formal diagnostic procedures and psychological testing) can be useful as part of a forensic evaluation. However, the key to a forensic evaluation is the emphasis on history.

We have somewhat artificially separated the types of assessment that clinicians would use depending on whether they were working for the defense or the plaintiff. Ideally, there should not be a difference between the two types of evaluations. And in fact, "objective" evaluations for the defense and the plaintiff should be rather similar in structure. Nevertheless, there are somewhat different agendas for the two sides. Furthermore, some aspects of any evaluation are inclusionary and some are exclusionary. For instance, ascertaining the presence of intrusive experience is more of an inclusionary task. Determining that the patient has never had a good work history is a relatively exclusionary task. We have tended to place the inclusionary tasks as part of the agenda of the plaintiff's evaluation and the exclusionary tasks as part of the defendant's evaluation. It is important to recognize, though, that a thorough evaluation (for the defendant or the plaintiff) will include both aspects.

The Agenda of the Plaintiff. Obviously, the agenda for the plaintiff is to determine whether or not the patient is having psychological difficulty as a result of the trauma. In order to determine this an evaluation needs to assess several areas.

1. *A description of the trauma from the patient's viewpoint.* What happened? What was the emotional and cognitive experience of the person?
2. *A formal psychological or psychiatric assessment criterion, including a mental status exam.* Does the person meet the DSM-III-R criteria for PTSD, or depression, or adjustment disorder?
3. *Most importantly, a before trauma and an after trauma evaluation. Were any of the symptoms present after the trauma present before the trauma? How has the person's social and work-related functioning changed from pre-trauma to post-trauma? The evaluation should be quite specific.*
4. *How has the clinical picture changed over time?* In many circumstances, a person is evaluated some time after the trauma. Has the clinical situation remained static, improved or deteriorated? How has the person attempted to cope with the problem? How has the person not been able to cope?
5. *A history of previous illnesses, injuries and trauma.* How has the person handled previous difficulties? Has the person usually overcome adversity, or usually taken a sick role?
6. *General background history* including: drug and alcohol use, previous mental health problems, relationships with family members.
7. *An evaluation of other possible sources of the disorder* (see the agenda for the defense).

The Agenda of the Defense. The defense is most often looking for the following types of information:

1. The fact that this is a legitimate claim, so they know that it is better to settle sooner rather than later (not out of altruism, but out of cutting losses).
2. Does the person's "symptoms" impede the persons ability to function?
3. Have there been other traumas prior to or subsequent to the trauma in question that are causally related to the symptomatic position?
4. Are there other medical or psychiatric reasons why this person would be having these symptoms?
5. Has the treatment that has been provided focused solely on the PTSD or has the person used treatment to deal with other unrelated issues?
6. The reasonableness or effectiveness of the treatment
7. Evaluation of the significance of the findings. What does the language of the plaintiff's report really mean? Sometimes reports are written in psychological jargon. The attorney for the defense may need to know what the jargon means.

The key to a forensic evaluation of PTSD, especially for the defense, is the history. The reason it is most necessary for the defense is simple. In order to make a DSM-IIIR diagnosis of PTSD, all one has to do is demonstrate that the criteria have been met. However, there can be all sorts of contaminating variables, such as concurrent or intercurrent stressors, other than the identified one in the legal proceedings. More importantly, before one can claim damages for various losses, one needs to demonstrate that one had something to lose in the first place.

For instance, if the plaintiff is saying they cannot work effectively since the trauma (and the development of PTSD), it would be important to know whether or not the plaintiff could work effectively before the trauma. Therefore, even though the defense evaluation is going to pay particular attention to looking at the history, the wise and ethical plaintiff clinician ought to be doing the same thing. If for no other reason, it may save him or her a great deal of embarrassment in court.

The assessment should include the following areas of inquiry:

Work history: Particularly job ratings; length of employment. The most accurate method of gathering information would be to contact the employer directly.
Stressors occurring within 1–2 years prior to the trauma: If the plaintiff has had major losses prior to the trauma, it becomes somewhat less clear if the trauma itself is the only variable causing the suffering.

Stressors occurring after the trauma and prior to symptom formation: To the extent that there are intercurrent stressors, the degree of causality between the trauma and the emotional distress becomes less clear.

Major relationships: Has there been marital strife before the trauma? Did anyone file for divorce? Are there major family problems that may be contributing to the clinical picture?

Previous psychiatric history: Has the person ever been hospitalized? Have they sought therapy before?

Drug and alcohol use: One other drug to assess is whether or not there have been changes in caffeine intake.

Medication: What medications has the person been on since the trauma? Have there been changes in medications? Do the medications have known use including psychological side effects?

What is going well in the person's life? This fascinating line of questioning can provide a wealth of data. For, example, a patient may discuss how depressed he is and give appropriate symptomatology. The psychologist for the plaintiff may be satisfied with this information. The independent psychologist may ask the patient questions about his summer vacation. If the person reveals that he went to the beach, did some sailing and waterskiing, a somewhat different clinical picture is revealed.[16] Questions that are relevant include: What hobbies does the person have? What does the person do on the weekend? What did the person do on vacation?

Does treatment seem much longer than reasonable? If so, what is the nature of the treatment? Was the treatment appropriate for treating PTSD? Were non-trauma related issues discussed? The notes of the treating therapist would be important data.

Interpretations and Conclusions of the Evaluation

There are general types of conclusions that the independent examiner can make. These are:

1. The plaintiff is as disabled as the plaintiff's evaluation says.
2. (a) The plaintiff has PTSD, but it is not as severe as stated.
2. (b) The plaintiff has PTSD, but is functioning better than stated.
3. The plaintiff has PTSD, but there is significant evidence that there are other factors contributing to the problem in addition to the trauma.
4. The plaintiff has some disorder. However, it is either not significantly related to the trauma, or is only partially related to the trauma.
5. The plaintiff was dysfunctional to a certain degree before the

trauma, so that a percentage of post-trauma dysfunction is not due to the trauma.

6. The treatment offered was appropriate.
7. The treatment offered the plaintiff was either not efficacious or not relevant to the trauma to some degree.

PROBLEMS IN ASSESSMENT AND DIAGNOSIS

The assessment and diagnosis of PTSD is frequently difficult. Atkinson et al. (1982) and Blank (1985a, 1985b) have addressed the major issues contributing toward such difficulties. Although their focus is the Vietnam veteran patient, many of the points raised are directly applicable to other PTSD patient populations. The issues raised by Atkinson et al. (1982) and Blank (1985, 1985b) are:

- professional bias against PTSD as a valid diagnosis
- denial of diagnosis workability
- professional resistance to DSM-III criteria
- adverse interactional styles in claimants and examiners
- lack of corroboration of data
- the "silent" patient
- exaggeration and falsification of data
- intercurrent stress
- "either-or" diagnostic judgments
- the co-morbidity theory
- the impact on examiners

Each of these issues is discussed briefly.

Professional Bias

The professional bias against PTSD as a valid diagnosis is twofold. First, some mental health professionals feel that PTSD does not exist as a separate diagnostic entity (Horowitz, 1973). The removal of "gross stress reaction" from the DSM-I certainly contributed toward this bias (Blank, 1985a). Second, others feel that PTSD is so rare that the majority of so-called PTSD cases are, in fact, indicative of another (preexisting) disorder (Atkinson et al., 1982). These pitfalls can be overcome by having possible PTSD cases diagnosed by objective clinicians.

Denial of Diagnosis Workability

Although the number of mental health professionals who dispute the validity of PTSD is on the wane, negative attitudes towards the diagnosis persist. Blank (1985a) notes several common concerns:

- There is the feeling among some clinicians that the diagnosis is circular: A demonstration of a traumatic stressor is indicated, but the precise definition of such a stressor is difficult.
- It is sometimes argued that the inter-rater reliability for PTSD is too low to make it a workable diagnostic category.
- Given the propensity for some lawyers to use PTSD as a defense in criminal cases, and the fact that the Veterans Administration awards disability to veterans with PTSD, there is fear that the diagnosis will be misused.

To avoid these potential pitfalls Blank (1985a, 1985b) argues that traumatic stressors are, in fact, not too difficult to define (i.e., combat, wartime or concentration camp imprisonment, torture, severe vehicular or air crashes, overwhelming natural disasters, rape, devastating collapse of buildings or other structures, severe fires, assaults, being kidnapped or taken hostage, etc.), that inter-rater reliability is acceptable, and that the effective use of PTSD as a defense in criminal proceedings is far from certain. The discussion of the primary and secondary symptoms associated with PTSD, as well as an awareness of the subtypes course of the disorder also enhance the workability of the diagnosis (see Chapters 1, 2, and 3).

Resistance to DSM-III Criteria

There is the tendency among some clinicians not to maintain strict adherence to the criteria for PTSD as outlined in the DSM-III (American Psychiatric Association, 1980). The presenting picture is often one in which the patient appears to satisfy most of the required criteria, and hence gives the impression of a PTSD case. This difficulty may be overcome by procedures such as lengthening diagnostic interviews (or not deciding upon a final diagnosis until adequate data have been collected) and standardizing diagnostic methods.

Atkinson et al. (1982) note that "partial" PTSD (PTSD without full symptoms) is common in those who were engaged in or near combat in Vietnam. They note that some clinicians have subsequently diagnosed PTSD due to "their sense of moral responsibility for veteran as victim." Similar reactions may also be expected from those treating rape victims, survivors of major disasters, etc. Again, strict adherence to the DSM-III criteria for PTSD is recommended as a means of avoiding this pitfall.

Atkinson et al. (1982) also note that some patients present with sufficiently intense symptoms, but without the necessary stressor (these are referred to as "idiosyncratic" disorders). They note that the proper diagnosis may be a generalized anxiety, phobic disorder, or obsessional disorder. However, they add that a more detailed inquiry, or data which might surface later in therapy, may reveal significant stressors, thus justifying a diagnosis of PTSD at that time.

Yet another manifestation of a reluctance to adhere to the DSM-III-R criteria is the tendency of some clinicians to use data unrelated to the diagnosis of PTSD as "proof" of its presence. For example, substance abuse and interpersonal difficulties are often noted in patients with PTSD. This has led some to consider the presence of such data as evidence supporting the diagnosis of PTSD in the absence of sufficient data to make a DSM-III-R diagnosis. "We advise examiners that if violence, disturbed relationships, and alcohol and drug problems are not found together with the more fundamental features and symptoms of post-traumatic stress disorder, this diagnosis is not to be made" (Atkinson et al., 1982, p. 1120).

Styles of Claimants and Examiners

Certainly with Vietnam veterans suffering from PTSD, but also with other patient populations manifesting PTSD, adverse interactional styles are not uncommon. Needless to say this can make diagnosis a difficult undertaking. It has been suggested that in Veterans Administration institutions a flexible staff be selected to work with such patients and that clerical and professional personnel be trained to handle possible problems. It has also been suggested that national service organization representatives and social workers prepare veterans for what to expect (e.g., the resurfacing of painful emotions) as well as procedural and bureaucratic requirements (Atkinson et al., 1982). Similar procedures could be adopted by emergency rooms handling rape cases, mental health agencies responding to a disaster, etc.

Lack of Corroboration

Given the nature of the stressors involved with patients manifesting PTSD it is often difficult to obtain sufficient corroboration of data (e.g., unprosecuted rape by a family member). With some patient populations (e.g., Vietnam veterans) it is particularly difficult to secure pre-trauma data, especially pre-trauma personality characteristics and social functioning. Hence, clinicians are often forced to base diagnoses almost entirely upon the patient's story and reported symptoms. As a means of dealing with this problem Atkinson et al. (1982) have suggested that only a few examiners be utilized for diagnostic interviews in institutions which handle many PTSD patients (e.g., Veterans Administration facilities). In this way examiners may acquire sufficient experience with PTSD presentations to maximize clinical judgment as an efficacious diagnostic tool.

The "Silent" Patient

Many patients who manifest PTSD find it difficult to relate to, and trust, the clinician. This is particularly true when the stressors in question involve experiences such as rape, torture, death-camps, and traumatic war experiences. For many victims of trauma there is a "command that the victim remain silent about the episode" (Lister, 1982). Hence, such patients are not forthcoming with necessary data. Since sufficient time for developing basic trust and support is not always available for diagnostic purposes it is recommended that the diagnosis of PTSD not be made (Atkinson et al., 1982). Diagnosis of PTSD should only be made when the required symptom clusters are reported by the patient.

Exaggeration and Falsification

With exaggeration of data this pitfall would appear to be one which is particularly applicable to Vietnam veterans, victims of accidents in the workplace, and car accident victims claiming to have PTSD. As Sparr and Pankratz (1983) have noted, with war events now distant and symptoms largely subjective it is easy to simulate the clinical picture of PTSD. In addition, checklists of PTSD symptoms have been widely distributed to veterans, thus precipitating the possibility that a patient may know the criteria required for diagnosis well in advance of the interview (Atkinson et al., 1982). Similar difficulties may exist for the other patient populations who might gain monetarily from a positive diagnosis of PTSD. Falsification of data would appear to be a problem likely to appear in all patient populations manifesting PTSD. Hence Type I errors are engendered in some cases. Concern over perceived weakness and inability to cope, as well as the reluctance of many victims to talk about their experiences, may lead to falsification of data in the other direction (i.e., symptoms are minimized). This leads to the possibility of Type II errors in diagnosis.

To overcome these diagnostic difficulties Atkinson et al. (1982) and Sparr and Pankratz (1983) recommend:

- interviewing by clinicians experienced in the diagnosis of PTSD
- contact with parties other than the patient (i.e., spouses, families, etc.)
- a second evaluation by an experienced examiner
- corroboration of data, if at all possible

Clearly, clinical astuteness is crucial for securing the required data for a positive diagnosis with patients who are reluctant to discuss their traumas, or who are consciously withholding material.

Intercurrent Stress

The elapse of time between the experience of the traumatic event and contact with mental health professionals may be great. In this period patients may experience additional stresses, some of which may be major. Indeed, Vietnam veterans and rape victims manifest many personal and social difficulties following traumatization. Consequently, clinicians are faced with differentiating which stressor is responsible for the current clinical picture, and whether PTSD or an anxiety disorder is an appropriate diagnosis.

Atkinson et al. (1982) suggest focusing on the time course and content of symptoms as a means of avoiding this difficulty. PTSD is diagnosed if symptoms existed before later traumas but worsened during subsequent stress, or the content of reveries or dreams is directly related to the significant stressor. Here the secondary stressors served as triggers for the original trauma. In situations where it is important to know which of two sufficiently intense stressors is related to PTSD symptomatology (e.g., claims made to the Veterans Administration by Vietnam veterans) the content of reveries or dreams is used as a guideline. Clearly PTSD would not be diagnosed, despite the presence of a significantly intense stressor, should the patient fail to meet all the criteria for PTSD (e.g., many PTSD symptoms exist, but intrusions do not relate to the original trauma).

"Either-Or" Diagnoses

Atkinson et al. (1982) note that many clinicians exhibit "excessive diagnostic parsimony," and fail to diagnose PTSD when other clinical entities appear more pronounced (e.g., substance abuse, psychosis, etc.). This is not in accordance with proper diagnostic procedures as indicated in the DSM-III:

> On both Axes I and II, multiple diagnoses should be made when necessary to describe the current condition. This applies particularly to Axis I, in

which, for example, an individual may have both a Substance Abuse Disorder and an Affective Disorder. It is possible to have multiple diagnoses
within the same class (American Psychiatric Association, 1980, p. 24).

Hence it is suggested that all justifiable diagnoses on Axes I and II be
made. Specific symptoms can then be related to different disorders, and
a determination of which disorder is primary, and which secondary, can
be made.

The Comorbidity Theory

A bias similar, but opposite, to the above also exists. Blank (1985)
notes that with the wane of the predisposition bias a "theory of comorbidity" has arisen. Hence, there is a bias among some mental health
professionals that steers them away from diagnosing PTSD independent
of other disorders. "This view may lead to either dismissal of the condition as an epiphenomenon or attributing it, along with other concomitant psychopathology, to more general underlying mental dysfunction"
(p. 84). Blank (1985) argues that studies which support this view are not
generalizable since the samples usually consist of treatment-seeking patients and/or are restricted to a particular ethnic-cultural group.

Impact on Examiners

The examination of PTSD patients can be very stressful to clinicians. As Blank (1985) notes:

> PTSD is caused by contact between the individual and the darkest and
> most violent forces of human nature. War, murder, rape, floods, etc. take the
> victim over the edge of life into serious confrontations with death or uncon-
> trolled violence. Some individuals are thereby transformed and become,
> at some level, bearers of the traumatic experience. The [examiner] with
> whom they come into contact is thus inevitably exposed to war, rape, flood,
> etc. (p. 88).

Clearly, vivid reports of living conditions in death camps, atrocities
during the Vietnam war, and the brutality of assault and rape, not to
mention descriptions from other events sufficiently intense to cause
PTSD symptomatology, can seriously affect mental health workers. Possible outbursts of anger directed at the examiner only add to the
problem.

To counteract the very real effects of working with PTSD patients
Atkinson et al. (1982) suggest the following possibilities:

- Examination of patients possibly manifesting PTSD on only one
  day each week

- Examination of patients with less severe symptomatology in between examinations of PTSD patients
- Meeting regularly with collegues and consultants

In this way the impact of the patient upon the examiner is reduced, as is the very real possibility of examiner "burnout" with a concomitant reduction in ability to accurately assess PTSD.

SUMMARY

This chapter has reviewed the assessment procedures for the valid diagnosis of PTSD in both non-crisis and crisis situations. In addition, diagnostic differentials and pitfalls in the accurate diagnosis of the disorder have been discussed. Although the assessment and diagnosis of PTSD is frequently difficult, it is necessary for treatment planning purposes. In the past unrecognized or ignored PTSD was treated inappropriately, sometimes with disastrous results (Grinker & Spiegel, 1945). The current procedures outlined above, especially the utilization of psychophysiological assessment (if possible) and the awareness of various difficulties, contribute positively to the detection of PTSD and thus enhance the possibility of appropriate therapeutic interventions.

IV

Therapy

8

General Considerations

INTRODUCTION

The treatment of PTSD patients is difficult for a variety of reasons. Not only is the nature of the trauma problematic for the patient, it is also threatening to the therapist (Haley, 1978). As with much of the literature on PTSD, a disproportionate amount of attention has been given to the treatment of Vietnam combat veterans. Nevertheless, many of the difficulties faced by therapists treating veterans with PTSD are also faced by therapists treating victims of other traumas.

THERAPY SHOULD OCCUR SOONER RATHER THAN LATER

The central principles of this tenet are derived from Crisis Theory (Burgess & Baldwin, 1981; Caplan, 1961; Greenstone & Leviton, 1981; Lindemann, 1944). Crisis theory holds that individuals maintain a "reasonably consistant balance between affective and cognitive experience" (Burgess & Baldwin, 1981). This balance is usually referred to as homeostasis. Diruption of the homeostatic equilibrium leads to the emergence of negative affects and a reduction in cognitive efficency. Sufficiently severe stressors may become "emotionally hazardous situations" (Caplan, 1961). Any stressor that is severe enough to meet DSM-IIIR criteria for PTSD is certainly an emotionally hazardous event. The resulting stress leads to the employment of both conscious and unconscious coping processes and behaviors. As Burgess and Baldwin (1981) note:

143

At best, coping is the process of mastery of a particular problematic situation. At worst, coping behaviors serve primarily to a vulnerable sense of self
without mastery of the situation. (p. 26)

Failure of the usual repertoire of coping processes and behaviors results
in psychological crisis.

Although, crisis theory was not developed with PTSD strictly in
mind, the reader can see the many parallels. Let us return to Figure 4.1
(p. 48), and expand the pictorial metaphor.

The further a patient has gone down a path toward a pathological
resolution of the crisis, the more difficult it becomes to get that person
on a path toward a healthy resolution. One either needs to backtrack the
entire distance toward the original juncture or to cut a path through the
forest. Either way, the job is much easier the closer one is to the original
point of diversion. The allegory is supported by the common finding
that patients with acute forms of the disorder tend to have a better
prognosis. In patients with delayed or chronic PTSD, the prognosis is
more guarded, and the treatment more complicated.

THERAPY SHOULD BE BRIEF

The therapy should remain focused on the traumatic situation and
patients' reactions to the trauma. The central outcome goal of working
with patients with PTSD is to return them to their level of functioning
before the trauma occurred (Figley, 1988; Horowitz, 1986). This should
not be confused with restoring people to the exact same way they were
before the trauma. This is what the patient often desires. PTSD patients
have undergone a trauma that has shaken their world. Therefore, they
cannot go back *exactly* as they were before the trauma. They will need to
have some additional ego resources (Horowitz, 1986) or more flexible
behavioral and cognitive responses (Meichenbaum & Cameron, 1983) so
that they will be better able to respond to the stress of dealing with the
traumatic experience. It is hoped that patients will also be better able to
cope with future stresses.

To put it another way, following Figure 4.1, the goal is to help the
person to get off the trajectory toward a maladaptive resolution, and on
to the trajectory toward an adaptive resolution. However, the goal is not
to walk down the latter path with the person.

There are four strategies of therapy that can be seen in virtually all
of the different forms of therapy of PTSD. These are:

1. supporting adaptive coping skills (ego)
2. normalizing the abnormal

Table 8.1. Common Strategies in the Treatment of Post-Traumatic Stress Disorder[a]

Therapy type	Decrease avoidance	Ego support	Normalizing the abnormal	Attribution of meaning
Psychodynamic	Encourage catharsis; interpret defenses that make numbing necessary	Teach "dosing," relaxation, desensitization; supply structure	Education about numbing and intrusive cycles	Interpretation
Family	Encourage family to talk about the trauma	Mobilize family as a support network	Education about symptoms, family response to stress	Reframing; healing theory
Cognitive/Behavioral				
Flooding	Flooding image	Relaxation	Education about classical conditioning	*Implicit:* You can survive experiencing the scene
S.D.	In vivo exposure	Relaxation	Same	*Implicit:* You can survive experiencing the scene
Behavioral Rehearsal	Practice coping skills in imagined or real situation	Relaxation coping skills	Same	*Implicit:* Self-efficacy
S.I.T.	Any of above	Relaxation, self-talk; palliative coping skills; instrumental coping skills	Same	*Explicit:* Development of alternative meanings; *Implicit:* Self-efficacy
Hypnosis	Uncovering, abreaction	Relaxation, trance as resource, ego-supportive suggestions, recovery of resources	Dissociative experience as potentially useful hypnotic skills	Reframing; future orientation

[a]Virtually all therapies discuss with the patient that it is normal to have these reactions, given the fact that they have been traumatized.

3. decreasing avoidance
4. altering attribution of meaning

A summary of these strategies across different treatment modalities is presented in Table 8.1

EGO-SUPPORTIVE INTERVENTIONS

There are many ego-supportive aspects of therapy with PTSD patients. A positive therapeutic relationship is an essential aspect of developing a supportive environment. It is important to make the development of a therapeutic alliance the first primary task of treatment, especially if the patient is going to be asked to face painful memories and experiences. Many of the educative interventions that are designed to normalize a patient's experience will build a positive relationship. Providing patients with rationales for the upcoming interventions (Meichenbaum & Cameron, 1983; Veronen & Kilpatrick, 1983) tends to give patients a sense of control, which is highly supportive of normal functioning.

Horowitz (1986) has discussed the general principle of using uncovering and explorative interventions when a patient in a denial-numbing phase and using supportive interventions when the person is in an intrusive-repetitive phase. While not all authors agree with the "phase" terminology, the consensus treatment plan follows the same pattern. The goal is to keep the person in an optimum range, between excessive denial and excessive intrusive symptomatology. Ego supportive interventions are designed to achieve one of several goals:

1. Reduce aversive symptoms (in order to break a negative feedback loop).
2. Provide sufficient resources to cope with resolution of trauma.
3. Increase adaptive functioning.

A given intervention can be used for multiple purposes. There are numerous specific inteventions that are used for support, some of these include: reducing external demands and rest (Horowitz, 1986); relaxation training, systematic desensitization, imagery, self-talk (Meichenbaum & Cameron, 1983), hypnotic retrieval of resources (Gilligan & Kennedy, in press), hypnotic ego-supportive suggestions (Brende, 1985) and medication (Horowitz, 1986, Roth, 1988).

DECREASING AVOIDANCE

Virtually all of the therapeutic approaches that will be discussed have avoidance reduction as a central treatment strategy. Avoidance can occur on a number of levels:

1. avoidance of affect/feelings (numbing)
2. avoidance of knowledge of event (amnesia)
3. behavioral avoidance (phobic responses)
4. avoidance of communication about the event

The tendency to avoid dealing with the trauma and its ramifications must be short circuited for two reasons. First, patients cannot process the traumatic experience itself if they avoid everything about it. Therefore, the experience remains toxic. Second, the avoidance itself becomes a secondary problem that further exacerbates the situation. For instance (as discussed in Chapter 6), the avoidance can generalize; it can lead to breakdown in communication between family members, and so on.

Psychodynamic, group, and family therapies encourage abreaction, catharsis, and vivid talking about the trauma and the feelings associated with it. Hypnotic therapies also utilize catharsis and abreaction. Cognitive-behavioral therapies often involve in vivo or in vitro exposure to traumatic analogues. In clinical practice there is often a great deal of overlap. For instance, in cognitive-behavioral therapy there is a degree of talking about the problem. In family therapy, a patient may be asked to do certain behavioral tasks that are like in vitro exposure.

NORMALIZING THE ABNORMAL

By definition, individuals who are suffering from PTSD have experienced an abnormal event. They experience reactions about which they have little understanding. Each of the therapeutic systems that will be described, explicitly or implicitly, help patients recognize that many of their reactions are normal, given the circumstances. Examples include: explaining the normality of returns of intrusive experiences after periods of calm (Horowitz, 1986), describing normal fear reactions (Veronen & Kilpatrick, 1983), dissociative phenomena as potentially useful hypnotic experiences (Gilligan & Kennedy, in press). The two purposes of these strategies are:

1. Prevention of further traumatization of the patients by their symptoms (in other words helping to inhibit a negative deviation amplification circuit;

2. Creating an atmosphere for patients to have an opportunity to utilize their own resources (that they might otherwise not use).

Interventions that center on normalizing the abnormal tend to involve facets of ego-supportive interventions as well aspects of interventions for altering the attribution of meaning.

ALTERING THE ATTRIBUTION OF MEANING

Since the attribution of meaning of the traumatic event, as well as one's responses to the event, is such an integral part of the disorder, it is not surprising that one of the common therapeutic strategies is to alter the meaning that is given to the traumatic event and its sequelae. For some of the models (stress-inoculation training, family therapy, hypnosis, psychodynamic) there are explicit interventions for helping patients change the meaning they have given to the traumatic experience. Some of these interventions include interpretation (Horowitz, 1986), reframing (Figley, 1988; Gilligan & Kennedy, in press), developing a healing theory (Figley, 1988); cognitive restructuring (Meichenbaum & Cameron, 1983), shifting attentional focus from the past to the future (Gilligan & Kennedy, in press; Veronen & Kilpatrick, 1983).

Implicit admonitions for attributional change exist in all therapeutic schools. The central themes are that the patient can survive experiencing the painful memories and emotions; the development of self-efficacy; and changing the self-image from passive victim to active survivor.

Frederick (1985) has defined one other attributional shift as the sine qua non for effective resolution of PTSD that is best categorized as supraordinate to all others. The goal of all therapy with PTSD patients is to generate the experience of "trauma mastery." Perhaps it is best to categorize the experience as the final common pathway to which all other interventions converge. The individual who successfully negotiates a traumatic experience has the attribution of meaning, " A terrible thing befell me. Not only have I survived it, but I have incorporated it into me. I may hurt more, but I am wiser or stronger. I have overcome the darkness and the pain. I can move forward in my life. I can laugh and love and work. I overcame the trauma; it did not overcome me."

RECURRING PROBLEMS IN TREATMENT

There are many difficulties involved in the treatment of patients with PTSD. Generally, these problems become more apparent as the magnitude of the trauma rises, as the chronicity of the disorder increases, or as the delay of treatment lengthens. Many of these hindrances have been mentioned earlier, albeit indirectly. Primary and secondary symptoms of the disorder that have become entrenched can present significant obstacles (see Chapters 2, 3). Problems in the assessment process, especially those which reside in the mental health care provider, also disrupt the treatment of patients with PTSD (see Chapter 7, pp. 134–139). Frequently noted *patient-based* difficulties with Vietnam veterans (Egendorf, 1978; Horowitz, & Solomon, 1978) that may be common in other types of PTSD include:

- the patient's reluctance to communicate with the therapist
- fearfulness that no one will truly understand the traumatic experience
- profound difficulty with interpersonal relations
- resentment towards authority figures
- powerful transference reactions
- substance abuse
- intense psychic numbing
- impaired self-concept
- pervasisve guilt and shame
- fears of losing control

Frequently noted *therapist-based* difficulties with Vietnam veterans (Egendorf, 1978; Haley, 1978) that may be common in other types of PTSD include:

- seeing patients as "villains" or as responsible for the trauma
- seeing patients as "victims"
- confusing (and equating) PTSD with compensation neurosis
- difficulties confronting one's own sense of vulnerability
- searching for the "fatal flaw" in the patient (which explains his/her succumbing to the trauma, and which would not relate to one's self)

SUMMARY

Because PTSD is generally regarded as a difficult condition to treat, multiple treatment modalities are often employed. These models will be presented in the following chapters. This chapter has been dedicated to delineating the common threads that traverse the different therapeutic modalities in treating persons suffering the results of trauma. The pattern that emerges as a result of keeping these common goals in mind can guide the clinician in several ways. It will help clinicians:

1. form an overall framework for treating patients with PTSD
2. design an integrated treatment plan, using different modalities
3. generate individualized (and/or new) treatment interventions for the special needs of a given patient
4. avoid common problems and mistakes in treating PTSD

9

Dynamic Psychotherapy

INTRODUCTION

A number of authors have argued against psychoanalytically oriented therapy for patients with PTSD (Figley, 1978; Fuentes, 1980; Walker & Nash, 1981; Haley, 1985). However, Horowitz (1973, 1974, 1976) advocates a dynamic approach to treatment, which he variously describes as "phase-oriented treatment," "focal psychodynamic treatment," "brief dynamic therapy," or "crisis-oriented psychodynamic therapy." What separates Horowitz's (1973, 1974, 1976; Horowitz & Solomon, 1975, 1978; Krupnick, 1980) approach to treatment from traditional psychoanalytic approaches is its pragmatism and synergy with information processing theory and cognitive approaches to emotion.

Another important factor inherent in Horowitz's (1973, 1974, 1976) approach is that it is not, like most other reports on treatment of PTSD, focused exclusively on Vietnam veterans. Indeed, his focus has been on victims of crime (e.g., rape, assault, robbery, etc.), accident victims, victims of traumatic loss, etc. Thus, it has a wide applicability to a variety of PTSD patient populations. In addition, Horowitz's (1973, 1974, 1976) approach provides a conceptual model within which to place other treatment strategies and applications.

THEORETICAL ORIENTATIONS

Building on classical and contemporary psychoanalytic theories of trauma, Horowtiz (1974) places central focus on information overload and incomplete information processing ("information" includes ideas from inner/outer sources, images, and affects). In essence, traumatic experience is too powerful to be immediately processed. It is therefore shunted out of awareness where it remains in storage in "an active form of memory." Denial-numbing protects the ego from the traumatic information. Frequently, intrusions (i.e., ideas, images, "attacks of emotion," compulsive behaviors, revivification, etc.) occur, often stimulated by external events. The oscillation of denial-numbing and intrusions continues until the information is fully processed; This is a natural aspect of information processing (Horowitz & Wilner, 1976). The focus is on completing the processing of information rather than abreaction and catharsis. Horowitz (1974) sees intrusions as potentially facilitating information processing, and defensive operations as promoting the gradual assimilation of traumatic experience. Maladaptive aspects also exist (intrusions can overwhelm patients and defensive maneuvers can hinder processing).

Following the above, Horowitz (1974, 1979, 1986) outlines progressive stages in the reaction to massive stress:

- *Phase I:* massive stress→crying out/stunned reaction
- *Phase II:* avoidance (denial and numbing)
- *Phase III:* oscillation period (denial-numbing↔intrusions)
- *Phase IV:* transition ("working through")
- *Phase V:* integration ("completing the processing of information")

Horowitz (1974) emphasizes that the processing and integration of traumatic experience is difficult.

PROCEDURES

The central thesis of Horowitz's (1973, 1974) approach to the treatment of stress disorders is the necessity of complete information processing (rather than character modification), with a dual focus on denial-numbing and intrusion phenomenon. The oscillation of the denial-numbing and intrusive apsects of the response to stress forms the basis for general stratagems of treatment. Horowitz's (1973, 1974) focus on character style (i.e., obsessive and hysterical) provides specific treatment approaches for various types of patient.

ASSESSMENT

Assessing the patient involves attendance to functional and/or dysfunctional defensive functioning. Horowitz (1973) approaches this in terms of "relative overcontrol" (i.e., strong tendencies for repression, denial, numbing, etc.) and "relative undercontrol" (i.e., a failure of defensive functioning with concomitant intrusions). He also examines the patient's overcontrol/undercontrol in relation to various psychic systems, namely, perception and attention systems, conscious representation, ideational processing systems, emotional systems, somatic systems, and control systems. These are illustrated in Table 9.1. An understanding of a patient's difficulties in terms of overcontrol and undercontrol within various psychic systems indicates various appropriate treatment techniques. Horowitz (1973) notes that, "In actual occurrence, the person might be in oscillation between overcontrol and undercontrol or in one state regarding a given ideational-emotional complex and another regarding a different ideational-emotional complex" (p. 511).

Table 9.1. Organization of Stress Responses as Related to States of Overcontrol and Undercontrol[a]

Systems	States	
	Relative Overcontrol	Relative Undercontrol
Perception and attention systems	Blunting of perceptions and attention (e.g., daze, selective inattention)	Hypervigilance, startle reactions
Conscious representation	Amnesia (complete or partial) and nonexperience	Intrusive-repetitive thoughts and behaviors (e.g., illusions, pseudo-hallucinations, nightmares, reenactments, ruminations)
Ideational processing systems	Denial, loss of reality appropriacy, constriction of associational width, inflexibility of organization of thought	Overgeneralization, inability to concentrate, preoccupation, confusion, disorganization
Emotional systems	Numbness	"Emotional attacks"
Somatic systems	Tension-inhibition symptoms	Chronic fight-flight sequelae
Control systems	Insufficiency of controls→activation of other symptoms (e.g., withdrawal, substitutive/counterphobic behaviors, alternating states of consciousness, regression)	

[a]Adapted from Horowitz (1973).

GENERAL STRATAGEMS OF TREATMENT

Horowitz's (1973, 1974) pragmatic approach to treatment follows a classification of treatment strategies based upon the prevalence of denial-numbing (overcontrol) and/or intrusion-repetition (undercontrol) with respect to controlling processes, information processing, and emotional processing.

Changing Controlling Processes

With respect to patient's in a denial-numbing phase, Horowitz (1973, 1974) includes:

- reducing controls (e.g., interpretation of defenses, hypnosis and narcohypnosis, suggestions, social pressure, psychodrama)
- changing attitudes making control necessary
- uncovering interpretations

With patients in an intrusive-repetitive phase, the following are classified as aiming at changing controlling processes:

- the supply of external controls (e.g., providing structure)
- assumption of ego functions by therapist (i.e., organize information)
- reduction of external demands and stimuli
- rest and relaxation
- providing identification models (e.g., through group membership)
- behavior modification

The goal of these interventions is not to increase or decrease controls, but to facilitate information processing.

Changing Information Processing

With respect to patients in a denial-numbing phase Horowitz (1973, 1974) includes:

- encouraging abreaction
- encouraging association, speech, the use of images in recollection and fantasy (not just words) enactments (e.g., role playing, psychodrama, art therapy)
- utilization of reconstructions (to "prime" associations and memory)
- maintenance of environmental reminders

With patient's in an intrusive-repetitive phase the following are appropriate interventions:

- working through and reorganization (e.g., through clarification, educative-interpretative work, etc.)
- reinforcing contrasting ideas
- removal of environmental stimuli
- the use of medication to suppress thinking

Again, the goal is to further the processing of the traumatic information.

Changing Emotional Processing

For patients in the denial-numbing phase the techniques Horowitz (1973, 1974) includes are: catharsis to counteract numbness and relationship building (with a focus on emotional involvement). For patients in the intrusive-repetitive phase, the following are appropriate: (1) support; (2) evoking contrasting emotions; (3) the use of medication to suppress overwhelming emotions; (4) desensitization procedures, and (5) relaxation and biofeedback. Not surprisingly, changing emotional functioning is often crucial.

GOALS, PHASES, AND PRIORITIES OF THERAPY

Horowitz (1973) notes that a shift in technique is required as the patient progresses through the various phases of treatment. Shifts in priorities and treatment goals mirror the changes in technique.

Priority I. When the patient is experiencing an external stress event, the treatment goals include (1) Protecting the patient; (2) removing the patient from exposure to the event; and (3) terminating the external event.

In essence, the impact of the stressor is reduced or eliminated. In situations of war this may include removing the patient from the front lines. However, in most cases the stressing event will have been terminated prior to treatment.

Priority II. When the patient is experiencing swings from denial-numbing to intrusion-repetition at intolerable levels, (1) Attempts are made to reduce the amplitude of the oscillation to tolerable levels; (2) support (emotional, ideational) is given; and (3) appropriate techniques are selected and applied (see above).

Priority III. When a patient is "frozen" in either a denial-numbing phase or an intrusive-repetition phase the therapist must aid in the proper "dosing" of the experience, that is, help the patient divide the experience into suitably small and therefore potentially integrated units of information. Again, appropriate techniques noted above are utilized.

Priority IV. When the patient is able to tolerate episodes of intrusion-repetition the patient goal becomes "working through." Detailed conceptual, emotional, object-relations, and self-image implications of the traumatic stressor are addressed.

Priority V. Termination is initiated when the patient appears able to "work through" ideas and emotions related to the event.

Horowitz (1973) cautions that different "complexes" (i.e., different information associated with different aspects of the original stressor) may progress independently of one another, making for a complex clinical picture. The therapist must attend to this resulting complexity in presentation.

TREATMENT OF PATIENTS WITH HYSTERICAL STYLES OF INFORMATION PROCESSING

Following Shapiro (1965), Horowitz (1974) characterizes the hysterical style as encompassing global attention, unclear/incomplete representations of ideas/feelings, partial/unidirectional associational lines, attention-seeking behaviors, fluid changes in mood/emotion, inconsistent attitudes, repetitive/stereotyped/impulsive relationships, and a dramatic life-style. Horowitz (1974) classifies the hysteric's cognitive maneuvers to avoid unwanted ideas:

- avoid representation
- avoid intermodal translation
- avoid automatic associational connections; avoid conscious problem-solving thought
- change self-attitude from active to passive (and reverse)
- alter state of consciousness (i.e., alter hierarchy of wishes/fears, blur reality/fantasy, dissociate conflicting attitudes, remove self as instigator of thought/action, etc.)

To aid the hysteric patient in completing the task of infomation processing of a traumatic event, Horowitz (1974) provides therapeutic tactics for various stylistic "defects" as they relate to various psychic functions (i.e., functions of perception, representation, multimodal translation, association, and problem-solving). These include:

- asking for details when the patient presents with global/selective inattention (perception function)
- encouraging abreaction/promoting reconstruction when images of others are impressionistic rather than accurate (representation function)
- encouraging the patient to talk (and providing verbal labels) when the patient's ability to translate images/enactions into words is limited;
- encouraging production/repeating the patient's words/enhancing clarification when inhibitions and misinterpretations interfere with the patient's association functions
- interpretations/maintenance of focus on topic when the patient "short-circuits" problem-solving;
- providing support when topics avoided due to the overwhelming nature of emotions (problem-solving function)

The above are all variations on clarification, the overarching therapeutic variable to be used with hysteric patients attempting to process traumatic information.

TREATMENT OF PATIENTS WITH OBSESSIONAL STYLES OF INFORMATION PROCESSING

Again following Shapiro (1965), Horowitz (1974) views the obsessive style as incorporating detailed/sharp attention to details, clear representations of ideas, meager representations of emotion, shifts in organization/implication of ideas (rather than following an associational line), avoidance of completion/decision-making, doubt/worry, productivity and/or procrastination, single-mindedness, intellectualization, tension, rigidity, routine interpersonal relationships, and dominance of superego dictates. To facilitate the processing of traumatic information in the obsessive style, Horowitz (1974) suggests:

- asking for overall impressions to counter overly detailed and factual perception
- asking about emotional experiences
- linking emotional meanings to ideational meanings to counter the isolation of ideas from emotions (representation function)
- focusing attention on images and felt reactions rather than on ideational aspects of information (translation of images to words function)
- interpretation of defensive operations when patient shifts set of meaning back and forth (association function)

- interpreting procrastination with endless rumination (problem-solving function)

The guiding principle in the treatment of obsessional types with stress-reponse syndromes is helping the patient focus long enough on a given piece of information so that its emotional facet may be unearthed, labeled, and integrated. This sustained attention facilitates information processing. The therapist achieves this focus by proceeding at a slower pace than the patient and emphasizing the concrete, rather than the abstract.

EFFECTIVENESS

For the most part Horowitz's (1973, 1974) papers are theoretical in nature. Treatment outcomes are not reported. However, Krupnick (1980), a coworker with Horowitz, reports success using insight-oriented brief psychotherapy with rape victims. Reports of increased feelings of control, confidence, assertiveness, and willingness to take risks were reported by those who completed a 12-session therapy. More positive self-images were also reported.

10

Behavioral Treatment

INTRODUCTION

The behavioral treatment of PTSD is, in most cases, the treatment of choice, particularly with patients manifesting PTSD, chronic or delayed. It is the only treatment modality that is supported by objective measures of success. Although the use of behavioral techniques is indicated for the treatment of traumatic memories, they need not be used entirely independently. Indeed, behavioral treatment of PTSD symptomatology is conducted only in the context of a supportive therapeutic alliance.

THEORETICAL ASSUMPTIONS

From a behavioral perspective it is the patient's response to memories of traumatic events that produces the primary manifestations of PTSD (Keane et al., 1985). It is further assumed that secondary features of the disorder are also, directly or indirectly, caused by the patient's reactions to his/her memories. Hence, the patient's memory of the original trauma(s) is (are) the focus of a behaviorally oriented approach to PTSD. A more extensive behavioral model of PTSD is described in Chapter 6.

Four major behavioral methods for the individual treatment of PTSD have been discussed in the literature. These include (1) implosive therapy/imaginal flooding; (2) systematic desensitization; (3) behavioral rehearsal; and (4) stress inoculation training. Each of these is briefly outlined below.

IMPLOSIVE THERAPY/IMAGINAL FLOODING

The most common form of behavioral treatment advocated in the literature is implosive therapy, or imaginal flooding. "Implosive therapy consists of the repeated imaginal presentation of [the patient's] traumatic event until the scene no longer evokes high levels of anxiety (extinction through exposure)" (Keane et al., 1985, p. 277). The goal of this procedure is to reduce avoidance of the traumatic memories and the anxiety caused by recollection.

Procedure

Various procedures for the use of implosive therapy with PTSD patients have been described in the literature (e.g., Keane & Kaloupek, 1982; Fairbank & Keane, 1982; Keane et al., 1985). The specific format for imaginal flooding advanced by Keane et al. (1985) is an adaptation of the technique developed by Stampfl and Levis (1967). Three stages are conceptualized.

- *Stage I:* relaxation training
- *Stage II:* pleasant imagery training
- *Stage III:* implosive therapy (imaginal flooding)

Stage I: Relaxation Training. The PTSD patient is taught a form of progressive muscle relaxation (Bernstein & Borkovec, 1973). As adapted by Keane et al. (1985) the patient first learns relaxation through the tension-relaxation of 16 muscle groups; then the tension part of the process is dropped, and finally cue-controlled training pairs cue words (e.g., "heavy, loose, and warm") to the relaxation response. Practice at home is encouraged. Relaxation training promotes the patient's ability to imagine a scene and enhances the reduction of anxiety following presentation of a traumatic scene in Stage III. Relaxation training generally takes about four sessions.

Stage II: Pleasant Imagery Training. Following the acquisition of the relaxation response the patient is taught to imagine pleasant imagery (following Lang, 1977). The rationale for this is twofold: pleasant imagery enhances relaxation and permits the therapist to determine the patient's capacity for imaginal work.

Stage III: Implosive Therapy. This stage is comprised of a number of subphases.

- developing a hierarchy of traumatic memories
- rating memories for stress
- relaxation
- setting the scene
- presenting traumatic cues
- presenting additional cues
- termination of scene
- ending session (with relaxation)

Developing a Hierarchy of Traumatic Memories. The patient is asked to identify his/her traumatic memory/memories. If there is more than one traumatic experience, the different traumas should be arranged hierarchically, from the least anxiety-provoking memory to the most. If there was just one trauma with multiple scenes, then a hierarchy of scenes can be constructed.

Rating Memories for Stress. On a scale of 1 to 10 each memory is rated (1 = not anxiety-provoking, 10 = most anxiety-provoking) in terms of subjective stress. With more than one memory, the one with the lower rating is addressed first in therapy.

Relaxation. Prior to the presentation of traumatic memories in sessions, the patient is encouraged to relax using his/her progressive muscular relaxation (PMR) skills. This enhances the patient's ability to imagine, and decreases thoughts unrelated to the task at hand.

Setting the Scene. Once the patient is relaxed the therapist uses sensory cues (visual, auditory, tactile, and olfactory) to create the scene of the trauma in the patient's imagination. Interaction with the patient about the details of the scene facilitates the most realistic image in the patient's mind.

Presenting Traumatic Cues. Following the setting of the scene the therapist guides the patient through the traumatic event. Keane et al. (1985) stress that this must be done supportively. Again, constant interaction with the patient permits the details of the event to be maximally imaged. The most anxiety-provoking factors of the incident are emphasized and prolonged.

Presenting Additional Cues. Keane et al. (1985) also aid the patient in remembering two additional cue categories. Following Lewis (1980), "reportable, internally elicited cues" and "hypothesized cues" (unre-portable cues hypothesized to relate to reportable, internally elicited cues) are used in this method of implosive therapy. "Reportable, inter-nally elicited cues are the patient's aversive thoughts, feelings, or images which are associated with the traumatic event. These cues represent the patient's cognitive reaction to the event and may include such feelings as guilt, anger, and grief" (p. 280). Hypthesized cues include: fear of bodily injury, fear of dying, fear of aggressive behavior, pubnishment for wrongdoing, and fear of rejection (Levis & Hare, 1977). It is argued that hypothesized cues are related to higher order conditioning to the original trauma, and thus promote many of the patient's difficulties (e.g., interpersonal difficulties, fears of exploding violently, fears of rejection, etc.).

Termination of Scene. Throughout the flooding procedure the ther-apist asks for subjective measures of distress using the 1–10 scale. Pro-longed exposure to the scene generally results in a decrease in rating; reduction over several sessions indicates a reduction in anxiety to that memory. In situations with more than one traumatic memory the next traumatic event on the hierarchy is only approached once anxiety has been reduced to the less anxiety-provoking event.

Ending Session. Relaxation is used again at the end of the session. A discussion of the session may also follow.

The amount of time required for reducing the anxiety caused by traumatic memories is determined by the rate of progress through the hierarchy. Each traumatic memory is attended to until the level of anxi-ety elicited remains low.

Effectiveness

Keane and Kaloupek (1982) document the efficacy of imaginal flooding through the course of treatment of a single patient, a Vietnam veteran with PTSD. Self-monitored data (i.e., hours of sleep, anxiety ratings, state anxiety measurement), performance on a standard psy-chological test, and physiological (i.e., heart rate) responses during scene presentation provided empirical, objective evidence for treatment efficacy. A 12-month follow-up supported long-term effectiveness. In a similar study of two Vietnam veterans with PTSD, Fairbank and Keane (1982) demonstrate the effectiveness of imaginal flooding using subjec-tive units of distress measures (SUDS) and physiological data (i.e., skin conductance responses and heart rate). Similar results for flooding are noted by McCaffrey and Fairbank (1985) with two patients, one a Vietnam veteran, the other a victim of four car accidents. Self-monitoring data (an 11-point fear thermometer) and physiological data (i.e., heart rate and skin response levels) confirmed the efficacy of the flooding procedure.

The two central problems with the outcome research are (1) they are case studies or small N studies; (2) they are using population samples of Vietnam veterans. Larger samples and more diverse population groups (e.g., rape victims, accident victims) and control groups would be helpful in evaluating flooding techniques.

SYSTEMATIC DESENSITIZATION

Systematic desensitization (SD) has been used to treat various symptom constellations commonly found with PTSD. Most of the literature in this area predates the diagnostic criteria of PTSD established in the DSM-III and relates specifically to the treatment of war-related experiences. However, it would appear to be applicable to all patient populations with PTSD.

Procedure

Three forms of SD have been suggested for treating PTSD related symptoms. These are (1) traditional SD; (2) individually administered *in vivo* SD; and (3) *in vivo* SD in dyads.

Traditional SD. Schilder (1980) notes the effectiveness of SD in treating a chronic recurring nightmare of a Vietnam veteran patient. He describes the nightmare as "a vivid reexperiencing of an extremely traumatic war experience." A first stage in therapy was teaching the patient relaxation techniques and encouraging pleasant imagery. A seven stage hierarchy was constructed based on the chronological events leading up to the trauma (witnessing the death of a fellow soldier who stepped on a land mine). The patient's anxiety increased as the dream progressed. Traditional SD (Goldfried, 1972) was employed, with additional self-administered SD at home. Treatment consisted of five biweekly sessions of 30 minutes' duration with a booster session two weeks after the termination of the first part of treatment.

Individually Administered **in vivo** *SD.* Kipper (1977) reports the use of *in vivo* SD with men suffering various fears resulting from war experiences. As with traditional SD, following the assessment procedures the patient was taught a standard relaxation technique and encouraged to practice this at home. A hierarchy of fears was then constructed. With one patient, a man suffering from a fear of seeing people bandaged, SD began in the office (a hierarchy was constructed in which the patient bandaged successively greater areas of the therapist's body). The next step is to encourage the patient to practice self-administered *in vivo* SD. The man with a fear of bandages was encouraged to walk through hospital wards and utilize his relaxation training; another patient with a phobic fear of noises hit a variety of objects each of which produced successively louder noises, and practiced relaxation techniques at each stage (he was also encouraged to tape-record the process and to listen to the procedure at home, again utilizing relaxation techniques).

In vivo *SD in Dyads*. This process follows the individually administered *in vivo* procedure above, except for the fact the hierarchies were worked through in pairs. Patients with different phobias were assigned to one another. Trials were followed by relaxation, and each item on the hierarchy was repeated until it no longer evoked anxiety (Kipper, 1977).

Effectiveness

Schilder (1980) notes successful treatment using traditional SD techniques. This is in accordance with other case study reports demonstrating the effectiveness of SD with recurring nightmares (e.g., Celluci & Lawrence, 1978). Kipper (1977) also reports success with individually administered *in vivo* SD and *in vivo* SD in dyads. In both studies success was defined in terms of a reduction of distressing symptoms and a maintenance of this reduction over time. McCaffrey and Fairbank (1985) included graded *in vivo* exposure (i.e., SD) to anxiety-provoking cues following flooding procedures. Objective data confirmed the effectiveness of *in vivo* SD treatment following flooding procedures. Once again, there is a need for larger samples, control groups, and different PTSD populations.

BEHAVIORAL REHEARSAL

Behavioral rehearsal has been used to treat a severe post-traumatic startle response with accompanying anxiety in the victim of a serious head-on vehicular collision (Fairbank, DeGood, & Jenkins, 1981). Although the patient in this case study was not reported as having the full symptomatic picture of PTSD, the authors note that post-traumatic startle responses are found in 34% of PTSD patients (Horowitz et al., 1980).

Fairbank et al. (1981) describe a two-phase treatment plan: relaxation training followed by behavioral rehearsal. The subject received three weekly sessions of progressive muscle and autogenic muscle relaxation, followed by use of tapes at home. Since the patient had had the accident on a two-lane highway and experienced startle responses only on similar roads, behavioral rehearsal consisted of driving on a practice course a mile in length on a heavily traveled two-lane highway. The practice course was driven twice daily for two weeks. Office visits were terminated after the fifth week of treatment.

Data for the behavioral rehearsal approach to the treatment of this patient with a post-traumatic startle response consisted in having the patient rate her level of anxiety (on a 1–5 scale) and record the number of startle responses per hour when driving on two-lane highways. These dependent measures were collected before treatment, during treatment, and after treatment at periods of one month, four months, and six months. Dramatic results were noted on both measures. Hence, the use of relaxation and behavioral rehearsal techniques for the treatment of persistent post-traumatic startle responses is an option.

STRESS INOCULATION TRAINING

Stress Inoculation Training (S.I.T.) was developed by Meichenbaum (1975) as an integrated approach to cognitive-behavioral therapy. Janis (1983) has described the underlying strategies of S.I.T. These include:

(1) "giving realistic information in a way that challenges the person's blanket immunity reassurances so as to make him aware of his vulnerability" and to motivate him to "plan preparatory actions for dealing with the subsequent crisis"; (2) counteracting "feelings of helplessness, hopelessness and demoralization" by calling attention to reassuring facts about personal and social coping resources that enable the person "to feel reasonably confident about surviving and ultimately recovering from the impending ordeal"; (3) encouraging "the person to work out his own ways of reassuring himself and his own plans for protecting himself." (pp. 71–72)

From a theoretical point of view, S.I.T.'s emphasis on developing a frame of reference of personal responsibility and activity for managing stressful events, with concomitant decreases in feelings of helplessness and decreases in attributions of passive-victimization suggest S.I.T. would be well suited for working with PTSD.

S.I.T. is broken into three phases: (1) conceptualization; (2) skills acquisition and rehearsal; (3) application and follow-through (Meichenbaum & Cameron, 1983). Table 10.1 shows the different procedures that can be utilized in each phase of treatment. These procedures are described more fully elsewhere (Meichenbaum, 1975; Meichenbaum & Cameron, 1983). The issues that are most relevant for the treatment of PTSD will be described.

In the conceptualization phase, education, as a form of collaboration, is emphasized. One of the factors that amplify PTSD symptoms is clients' expectations that they should not be having so much difficulty. As described previously, it is important to educate clients about the untenability of a blanket immunity response to trauma. In the data collection aspect of S.I.T., a particularly important approach is image-based reconstruction. Clients are asked to go back to the traumatic situation and visualize it in their mind's eye. The details of the covert images can lead to a more complete understanding of the cues, attributions, and idiosyncratic experiences that are important aspects of the trauma. The "images" should be as detailed as possible, including visual, auditory, kinesthetic and olfactory modalities. Internal self-statements, attributions, and evaluations provide crucial data for treatment.

Following Lazarus and Launier (1978), a distinction between instrumental and palliative coping skills is drawn in phase 2 of S.I.T.

> *Instrumental* coping refers to actions that serve to meet environmental demands or alter stressful situations and transactions. *Palliative* coping involves responding as adaptively as possible in unavoidable stressful situations when instrumental coping is not possible. (Meichenbaum & Cameron, 1983, p. 132)

This distinction is particularly significant because therapists, and more importantly, clients need to recognize that some pain and stress are simply unavoidable. In any cases the traumatic incident is over, and has a low probability of recurrence. Clients are left with symptoms for which there are few instrumental skills for coping. For instance, it is unreasonable for crime victims to *never* have intrusive memories of the experience or have moments of fear. The relevant issue is whether or not clients have *palliative* coping skills for those times. Examples of palliative skills include: reassuring self-statements and relaxation responses. An example of an instrumental coping skill for possible future violence would be learning karate.

Veronen and Kilpatrick (1983) report the use of S.I.T. with 25 rape victims. The training was targeted to ameliorate rape-induced fear and anxiety. In the first phase of treatment the rationale for S.I.T. is given to

Table 10.1. A Flowchart of Stress Inoculation Training[a]

Phase One: Conceptualization

(a) Data collection—integration
  - Identify determinants of problem via interview, image-based reconstruction, self-monitoring, and behavioral observation
  - Distinguish between performance failure and skill deficit
  - Formulate treatment plan—task analysis
  - Introduce integrative conceptual model

(b) Assessment skills training
  - Train clients to analyze problems independently (e.g., to conduct situational analyses and to seek disconfirmatory data)

Phase Two: Skills Acquisition and Rehearsal

(a) Skills training
  - Train instrumental coping skills (e.g., communication, assertion, problem-solving, parenting, study skills)
  - Train palliative coping skills as indicated (e.g., perspective-taking, attention diversion, use of social supports, adaptive affect expression, relaxation)
  - Aim to develop an extensive repertoire of coping responses to facilitate flexible responding

(b) Skills Rehearsal
  - Promote smooth integration and execution of coping responses via imagery and role-play
  - Self-instructional training to develop mediators to regulate coping responses

Phase Three: Application and Follow-Through

(a) Induce application of skills
  - Prepare for application using coping imagery, using early stress cues as signals to cope
  - Role-play (a) anticipated stressful situations and (b) client coaching someone with a similar problem
  - "Role-play" attitude may be adopted in real world
  - Exposure to in-session graded stressors
  - Use of graded exposure and other response induction aids to foster *in vivo* responding and build self-efficacy

(b) Maintenance and generalization
  - Build sense of coping self-efficacy in relation to situations client sees as high risk
  - Develop strategies for recovering from failure and relapse
  - Arrange follow-up reviews

General Guidelines for Training

  - Attend to referral and intake process
  - Consider training peers of clients to conduct treatment. Develop collaborative relationship and project approachability
  - Establish realistic expectations regarding course and outcome of therapy
  - Foster optimism and confidence by structuring incremental success experiences
  - Respond to stalled progress with problem-solving versus labeling client resistant
  - Include family members in treatment where this is indicated

[a]Reprinted from D. Meichenbaum and M. Jaremko, eds. (1983). *Stress Reduction and Prevention*. New York: Plenum.

the clients. Education about the classical conditioning model of rape-induced fear was offered. The women are educated about the normality of their responses, as well as the different ways in which fear and anxiety manifest themselves (e.g., behavioral, cognitive, and physiological). The phenomenon of the fear response occurring in stages, and not being all-or-nothing events is also discussed.

In the skill-acquisition phase of the training, each coping skill is taught in a standardized format.

> It includes a definition of the coping skill, the rationale and mechanism for the skill, a demonstration or explanation of the skill, and two applications of the skill. The first time the skill is applied, it is used with a non-target related fear; the second time, it is used with a target fear. (p. 360)

The skills include muscle relaxation, breath control, role-playing, covert modeling, thought stoppage, and guided self-dialogue. At the end of each session homework is given. The tasks are either "practicing a coping skill, confronting an everyday stressor, or completing an approximation of the target fear" (p. 363).

Ayalon (1983) describes a case of a crisis intervention approach based on principles of S.I.T. that was used after a terrorist attack in Nahariya with 54 children with symptoms of PTSD. The children were 8–14 years old, and were grouped according to age. The training was carried out in small peer groups.

The stages of treatment were (1) ventilation of feelings (verbal and nonverbal modalities were used); (2) abreaction through role-play and retelling of the events; (3) aggression channeling through the use of puppets and plays (the execution of the terrorists brought relief); (4) gradual *in vivo* exposure (gradual exposure to noises was carried out, using systematic desensitization procedures). Parents took the children to the beach where the terrorists had landed. The *in vivo* exposure was deemed more effective; (5) cognitive reappraisal of the experience by looking at their behaviors and reactions in light of retrospective knowledge; (6) working through was characterized by more structured activities, such as writing poems and erecting memorials; (7) mapping alternatives involved making suggestions for future encounters with danger based on all the current information. Follow-up at eight months found no perseverance of symptoms in all but a few children. Without a control group, it is difficult to know if the children would have improved without assistance.

However, Ayalon (1983) reported a natural experiment, where an ultrasonic boom sent an entire school into the air shelter. More than 400 children panicked as in previous attacks. However, there was one group of 50 children who remained calm and organized. These children had completed a course of coping training for shelling raids, and were equipped with alternative coping behaviors.

Anger and rage are often associated with PTSD. Some patients tend to act out these feelings, whereas other patients are quite frightened of the intensity of the affect. They experience a threat to their ability to control themselves. Novaco (1977) has reported successfully using S.I.T. for control of anger problems. Unfortunately, the use of S.I.T. for anger management has not been reported for patients with PTSD.

Effectiveness

All of the studies mentioned (Ayalon, 1983; Novaco, 1977; Veronen & Kilpatrick, 1983) have reported positive results. One noticeable trend is that S.I.T. appears to be the only behavioral intervention used in studies with large numbers of subjects. There is even an example of a quasi-experimental control group design.

In addition, Veronen and Kilpatrick (1983) have pointed out that, in many cases of rape-related PTSD, much of the symptomatology diminishes without treatment within three months. They emphasize the need for control groups when evaluating treatment paradigms for victims of recent trauma. The use of control groups is a much needed improvement in the methodology of outcome evaluation for all treatment paradigms.

Veronen and Kilpatrick's (1983) work also demonstrated that, when given a choice, both patients and therapists preferred S.I.T. to systematic desensitization or peer counseling. While these findings may be an artifact of experimental demand characteristics (Orne, 1969), they may indicate S.I.T.'s superiority to other behavioral interventions in diminishing treatment dropout.

11

Hypnotherapy
and Narcosynthesis

HYPNOTHERAPY

Theoretical Assumptions

Perhaps the symptom that is the sine qua non of PTSD is the reexperiencing of the event through intrusive imagery. The dissociative quality of these experiences (that is, the perceived nonvolitional aspect of the experience) was part of the unsuccessful impetus to place PTSD under the dissociative disorders in the DSM-III-R (Keane, personal communication, March 1988). Yet, some people who are traumatized develop PTSD, while others do not. Is it possible that people who develop PTSD are more hypnotizable than those who do not?

Stutman and Bliss (1985) separated 26 Vietnam veterans into high and low PTSD symptom groups. The veterans in the high-symptom group were found to be significantly more hypnotizable than those in the low-symptom group. Spiegel, Hunt, and Dondershine (1988) compared the hypnotizability, as measured by the Hypnotic Induction Profile (Spiegel & Spiegel, 1987), of 65 Vietnam veterans with PTSD with 83 normal volunteers and 115 patients with other types of psychiatric disorders (e.g. generalized anxiety disorder, affective disorders, and schizophrenia). Patients with PTSD were significantly more hypnotizable than normals and the other patient groups. As with previous work (Lavoie & Sbourin, 1980; Pettinati, 1982; Spiegel, Detrick, & Frischolz,

171

1980; Spiegel, 1980), the patients with other psychiatric disorders were less hypnotizable than normals.

This finding demonstrates that at least as far as hypnotizability is concerned, patients with PTSD are different than all other types of patients. For instance, the mean hypnotizability score of patients with generalized anxiety disorder was just about half that of the patients with PTSD. These studies also indicate the importance of dissociation as an underlying factor of PTSD symptomatology. The other implication from these studies is that hypnosis may be a particularly helpful type of therapy for PTSD.

Much of the literature on hypnotherapy and PTSD has emphasized the use of traditional hypnosis as well as psychodynamic explanatory principles (Brende, 1985; Brende & Bennedict, 1980; Silver & Kelly, 1985). Following an object relations model (see Chapter 6), Brende (1983, 1985) emphasizes the importance of "splits" in the personality as preventing the working through of the traumatic event. These splits (often identified via amnesias) prevent adequate "rehearsing of the past." The term "rehearsing of the past" is roughly equivalent to the cognitive processes discussed by Horowitz (1986) and Epstein (1990). Hypnotically induced abreaction is viewed as helpful in reintegrating the traumatic complexes and "healing the splits."

Hypnotic Procedures

Brende (1985) notes four ways in which hypnosis can be used:

- as a supportive technique (for controlling anxiety);
- as an uncovering technique (when the patient has amnesia for the trauma);
- as an abreactive technique (when the patient is symptomatic); and
- as an integrative technique (to heal splits in the psyche).

It is important to note that in clinical terms there is not such a clear dichotomy between these approaches. In any given session, and certainly across a treatment protocol, more than one approach will be used.

Hypnosis as a Supportive Technique. The use of hypnosis as a supportive technique enhances patients' capacity to control anxiety and other dysphoric experience, and may enhance their ability to trust the therapist (Brende & Benedict, 1980; Brende, 1985). It is best to frame the use of hypnosis as giving patients more control. In fact, one can offer the rationale to patients that some of their symptoms are due to the fact that they are already using hypnosis without knowing that they are doing so. Furthermore, they have a talent for using dissociation. In addition, it has been the fact that they did not know they had this talent nor did they know how to control it that has been part of the problem up to now. Finally, they can learn how to master the control of this talent for their own benefit. Quite often the response from patients is relief. One patient stated: "You are the only person that has ever given me a way to understand what is happening to me."

Basic hypnotic techniques include relaxation, guided imagery to safe places, general ego-strengthening suggestions. Self-hypnotic techniques can also be taught to patients. Hypnosis can be used in the context of individual or group treatment.

This basic use of hypnosis most frequently occurs at the onset of therapy to promote relaxation and an increased sense of well being. In this framework, hypnosis is usually viewed as a palliative intervention to make the patient feel more comfortable to talk or feel more trusting of others (Brende, 1985).

However, hypnosis can be viewed as much more than a palliative "salve" administered by the doctor to the patient. In more modern hypnotic frameworks, hypnosis is viewed as a cooperative venture between client and therapist (Araoz, 1985; Erickson & Rossi, 1979; Lankton & Lankton, 1983, 1987) that is truly supportive of the healthy functioning of the ego. Trance is used to retrieve intrapsychic resources that have been "lost" or have not been brought to bear on the traumatic experiences (Lankton & Lankton, 1983, 1987). Hypnosis is particularly useful for developing states of inner security (Gilligan & Kennedy, in press), useful dissociation and objectivity (Erickson & Rossi, 1979), feelings of power (Gilligan & Kennedy, in press; Lankton & Lankton, 1987), reorientation to the future (Erickson, 1948, 1954; Erickson & Rossi, 1979; Gilligan & Kennedy, in press). These resources once brought into the foreground can become powerful allies in the recovery from trauma.

Hypnosis as an Uncovering Technique. Once the patient has become comfortable with hypnosis, and has established a trusting relationship with the therapist, hypnotic techniques can be used to allow the patient to gain access to denied or repressed material. Brende (1985) notes that "specific target symptoms" such as pain or destructive dreams can be used as guides for the hypnotic work. For instance, a patient with bad dreams, while in hypnosis, can be invited to have the dream in a different manner that is less frightening and gives the patient and therapist more obvious information about what is bothering the patient. The process is construed as a "gentle opening-up" process. Once the person's associations are "opened up," either abreaction can be suggested, or a more gradual recovery of memory can be suggested.

Lankton (1988) has described one method used to help uncover the traumatic event for clients who are particularly phobic of the hidden event. The technique called "emanated image dissociation" asks that the client examine the trauma in fantasy. In actuality, the client does not consciously examine the event at all, at least at first. The client is hypnotized. Suggestions are given that (1) the client imagine an image of himself and that (2) the fantasized image recalls the traumatic event from a dissociated vantage point (e.g., on a movie screen). This can be repeated several times until the client is ready to watch the event without the intervening variable. In certain cases the double dissociation does not offer sufficient protection. In these cases, an additional image can be added. So the client sees image 1. Image 1 can see image 2 and image 2 can watch the trauma. Once the client is sufficiently desensitized, image 2 can let image 1 watch the trauma. Then finally the client, in a trance, can watch the trauma.

Hypnosis as an Abreactive Technique. Abreaction in the hypnotic context usually refers to the patient vividly reliving the traumatic event while in a trance. Brende (1985) describes the following issue: On the one hand, the recovery of the repressed material and reliving the incident has often been cited as important goals of hypnotic therapy. On the other hand, it has also been stated that the relief of symptoms from this technique has not been permanent.

It is not enough to just have the patient reexperience the trauma another time. The therapeutic difference in a successful abreactive approach is that the patient comes to make new meaning out of the old experience. This can happen in one of several manners. Brende (1985) quotes Jung (1954):

> The mere rehearsal of the experience does not itself posses a curative effect: the experience must be rehearsed in the presence of the doctor... (the patient's) conscious mind finds the doctor a moral support against the unmanageable effect of the traumatic complex. No longer does he stand alone in his battle with these elemental powers.... (pp. 132–133)

Thus, the first difference (as in all psychotherapy) is the therapeutic relationship. The difference is that the patient is not alone in the experience. Another manner in which to alter the revivified experience is by providing the patient with different hypnotically derived resources before the patient is regressed to the traumatic event (S. Lankton, personal communication, April 1988). As already mentioned, resources could include a sense of power, comfort with anger, or increased dissociation and objectivity. With the new and strengthened resources in the foreground the person can reexperience the trauma in a more controlled fashion.

For example, Silver & Kelly (1985) report a case of a Vietnam veteran who had extreme guilt because he believed that he had made mistakes that caused his patrol to be ambushed. He could not completely recall the actual combat experience. While in trance, he was asked to review the entire combat experience in an objective fashion. He discovered that even though he felt that he did something wrong, in fact he had made no serious errors.

Restructuring the Traumatic Incident. A related technique is to actively suggest that the patient use the new resource to reexperience the trauma differently. For instance, if the patient was raped, and was humiliated because she was afraid to fight back, the resources of anger and security could be developed. Then she could be regressed to the rape and reexperience it, only this time she would fight back and win.

A patient, whom one of the authors saw, had fallen from a ladder. He kept experiencing intrusive imagery of seeing a man fall from a ladder and land in a pool of blood. After hypnotizing the patient, it was suggested that he watch the scene again, only this time something different and less traumatic would happen. A number of possibilities were offered as well as the option for anything the patient could come up with. The man in the image disappeared. This was practiced a few times. The patient was then told to "try as hard as you can to see the image in the old way."[17] He could no longer produce the old image at will. The man kept disappearing. Posthypnotic suggestions were offered that it would be too hard to have the old image because the new one would interfere.

McMahon (1986) describes a technique of suggesting that patients imagine a part of themselves being a benign and caring parent who can intervene and help the younger traumatized self in some useful way. In some cases, the patient is afraid that he may be dead or will soon be dead. Symptom formation can develop around the need to know that one is alive. Mutter (1987) gives suggestions that patients will find alternative methods for knowing that they are alive.

Hypnosis as an Integrative Technique. Spiegel, Hunt, and Dondershine (1988) state:

> Trauma can be understood as the experience of being made into an object, a thing: the victim of someone else's rage, of nature's indifference, of one's own physical and psychological limitations. Along with the pain and fear associated with rape, combat trauma or natural disaster comes an overwhelming and marginally bearable sense of helplessness, a realization that one's own will and wishes become irrelevant to the course of events; this leaves a view of the self as damaged or contaminated by humiliation, pain, and fear that the event imposed.... (p. 304)[18]

In other words, the old experience of the self (as a self-efficacious subject who has control, will, options, and so on) is dissociated into the background (as if for safekeeping). The new foreground of the self is one that is damaged, helpless, fearful, and humiliated. This is the experienced state of affairs during an intrusive phase (Horowitz, 1986) of PTSD. During a numbing phase (Horowitz, 1986), the humiliated and damaged sense of self is dissociated in the background. In the foreground is a constricted, reconsolidated self that is constricted with the conscious or unconscious awareness that the self is now fragmented (Spiegel, Hunt, & Dondershine, 1988).

The reason that patients with PTSD split off or dissociate aspects of their experience is that they cannot cope with overwhelming experience (Horowitz, 1986), including the sense of the self as damaged and humiliated (Spiegel, Hunt, & Dondershine, 1988). Thus, the problem of experiencing the self as whole again involves the difficulty in keeping both the damaged self and the healthy self in the foreground at the same time.

The splits in the personality can take numerous forms. In Vietnam veterans Brende (1983, 1985) and Brende and McCann (1984) note "victim identification" (i.e., a "victim self"), "identification with the aggressor" (i.e., a "killer self") and a "protective self" (see Chapter 6). Dissociated aspects of the self can be linked to fear dehumanization, anger, rage, and guilt (Brende & Benedict, 1980). In several rape cases, we have noted a tendency for the split to come between the "helpless victim self" and the "powerful self." In these few cases, the problem appeared to be that the women's sense of power was contaminated by their rage at being raped. Therefore, the rage and the power were dissociated from the rest of the self.

Hypnosis can be used to facilitate the integration of split off parts of the personality. The general goal is for the patient to realize that each aspect of the self has value in and of itself; and furthermore, each part has value for the other parts. Part of the goal is for the patient to come to realize that it is the separation of the parts that is the most problematic aspect of their attempted solution.

> One story that one of the authors (RAS) just about always tells patients conveys this idea. It comes from a Star Trek episode where Captain Kirk is split into two Captain Kirks by a malfunctioning transporter. The one Captain Kirk is rational, good, and nice. The other Captain Kirk is irrational, angry, and frightened. The problem is that no matter how much the nice Kirk does not like the angry animal-like part of himself, without it he can not command the ship. The show ends with the nice/good Kirk recognizing the value of his darker side. The angry scared Kirk recognizes the value of nice Kirk by asking for help. Once reintegrated Captain Kirk can command again.

Lankton (1988) describes a second procedure that helps to bridge the barriers between the traumatized helpless experiences and normal states of consciousness usually associated with coping skills. In trance, clients are asked to organize their trance experience so that they feel an abundance of coping skills and resources. They can use any past, present, or fantasized experience that they would like. They are then asked to open their eyes while continuing to be aware of the resource feelings. Once this has been established, clients are asked to keep these resource feelings constant while they visually and auditorily experience themselves in the original traumatic situation. Nevertheless, their eyes are open; they are aware that they are in the therapy room and they have the experiences of the resource feelings. The goal of this approach is to help break down the dissociation between the traumatic state of consciousness and the state of consciousness normally associated with coping. "When bits and piece of the traumatic event are stimulated by the environment, clients will also find they experience feelings of resourcefulness and coping."

Hypnosis is not a panacea. It cannot be totally divorced from psychotherapy in general. It is often combined with more standard therapeutic procedures. Working through is an important aspect of the treatment (Brende, 1985; Mutter, 1987; Silver & Kelly, 1985). For instance, if a patient has difficulty following suggestions related to restructuring the trauma, it may be an indication that there are other factors besides the trauma itself at work. Mutter (1987) described the case of a man who was shot. He was given the suggestion that he see the assailant being bound and rendered helpless and under his control. It was also suggested that he see himself punishing the assailant. The patient could not comply with the second suggestion. Further exploration revealed that his father would beat him any time he showed aggression. Once the patient worked through the belief that the assault was a punishment for these repressed aggressive feelings the symptoms subsided.

Although they are addressing hypnotherapy of survivors of incest and not PTSD per se,[19] Gilligan and Kennedy (in press) specify several interesting issues for treatment consideration that are applicable for PTSD. First, they emphasize the importance of developing themes of mastery. For instance, the phenomena of intense memories (i.e., intrusive experience) it was framed as an important ability. If a person can have intense "bad" memories they can also learn to have intense "good" memories.

A second issue indirectly raised by the work of Gilligan and Kennedy (in press) is the use of hypnosis to work on multiple aspects of the client's problem, one piece at a time. Each weekly meeting worked on one mastery theme. Some of these themes included: accessing security and an inner center, envisioning a positive future, reclaiming the past: power symbols and other resources, body image, anger, secrets, sexuality, and generating altered states without substance abuse. The goal of this type of approach is to restore and strengthen the ego so that the individual is no longer overwhelmed by the trauma [as previously described by Spiegel, Hunt, and Dondershine (1988) on p. 8]. This approach is not hypnosis as magic. It seems very much akin to the methodical approach seen in Stress Inoculation Training (Meichenbaum, 1975).

One final issue that is partially raised by Gilligan and Kennedy (in press) is the emphasis they placed on helping their patients develop a future orientation. One of the problems of patients with PTSD is their tendency to look back instead of forward. Part of the working through process in psychodynamic therapy involves applying what is learned in the therapy sessions to daily living. In hypnotic therapy, it is equally important to link the newly learned experiences to patients' present and future social environments (Lankton & Lankton, 1983). It may be that part of the failures maintaining therapeutic success with traditional hypnosis was the inattention paid to this important aspect of therapy.

Indications and Contraindications

As a guide to deciding when each of these approaches is appropriate, Brende (1985) and Silver and Kelly (1985) recommend an assessment of a number of variables including (1) therapist familiarity/experience with hypnotherapy; (2) quality of the therapeutic relationship; (3) the patient's ego strength; (4) the patient's character defenses; (5) the patient's hypnotizability;[20] (6) phase of treatment; (7) degree of patient-therapist contact; (8) setting (e.g., inpatient vs. outpatient), and (9) therapeutic goals at the moment. In Table 11.1 we have presented some additional guidelines.

There are several significant contraindications for using hypnosis. The most important reason to avoid using hypnosis is when the therapist does not trust the patient. "Not trusting the patient" generally means that the therapist has no idea how the patient will respond[21] (S. Lankton, personal communication, April 1988). Hypnosis should only be used with borderline and psychotic patients after a therapeutic alliance has been achieved (Baker, 1986). In general, difficulties with hypnosis are reduced when permissive inductions are used, patients are given as much control as possible, and therapists are experienced with hypnosis.

Silver and Kelly (1985) have noted the advantages of hypnotherapy over drug-induced techniques (e.g., sodium amytal). These include:

- No anesthesiologist is needed.
- There is no concern with drug side effects or interactions.
- Hypnosis provides a finer control over how material is brought into awareness.
- Hypnosis provides a means of deciding which material is recalled.

Effectiveness

To date, all accounts of the successful use of hypnotherapy with patients suffering from PTSD have been anecdotal (Brende & Benedict, 1980; Brende, 1985; Silver & Kelly, 1985; Lankton, 1988; Mutter, 1987). The various case studies presented by these authors and the evidence of

Table 11.1. Guidelines for Hypnotic Techniques with PTSD

Variable	Type of Hypnotic Technique			
	Supportive	Uncovering	Abreactive	Integrative
Therapist familiarity/experience with hypnosis	Lower ⸻⸻⸻⸻⸻⸻⸻⸻⸻⸻⸻⸻⸻⸻⸻⸻ Higher			
Quality of therapeutic relationship	More tentative ⸻⸻⸻⸻⸻⸻ Less tentative			Variable[a]
Patient ego strength	Low-high	Medium-high	Medium-high	Low[b]-high
Patient defensive style	Intrusive	Denial	Intrusive or denial	Dissociated
Phase of treatment	Earlier ⸻⸻⸻⸻⸻⸻⸻⸻⸻⸻⸻⸻⸻⸻⸻⸻⸻⸻ Later			
Therapeutic goal	Symptom reduction of resource retrieval	Finding time/place of meaningful material	Retrieving the trauma itself/restructuring trauma	Healing splits in the personality

[a]Preliminary integrative work can be done to strengthen the therapeutic relationship. The more a person has splits in the personality the more important it is for the therapist to attend to the different parts. Aligning oneself too much with one of the sides, the more the other sides will exhibit resistance.
[b]Sometimes doing integrative work can strengthen a patient's ego functioning. However, this would probably be done without uncovering too much of the trauma at first, and emphasizing the usefulness of different parts in combination with supportive techniques.

higher hypnotizability in PTSD patients suggest the effectiveness of hypnotherapy, at least when applied by experienced hypnotherapists in appropriate situations. It would certainly be useful to have clinical studies with larger samples of patients with clear pre- and post-outcome variables.

NARCOSYNTHESIS

Although Kolb and Mutilipassi (1982) and Blanchard et al. (1982) refer to the therapeutic use of narcosynthesis in the treatment of PTSD, it is Kolb's (1985) description of the process that is the major contribution in the field.

Theoretical Assumptions

As with hypnotherapy, the central assumption underlying use of narcosynthesis is the effectiveness of catharsis in certain situations. More precisely, narcosynthesis has the potential of positively impacting upon massive repression. Kolb's (1985) orientation is psychodynamic.

Indications/Contraindications

Kolb (1985) describes the use of a single narcosynthesis session in the initiating phases of individual and/or group therapy. Indications for the use of narcosynthesis center upon the observation of recurrent behavioral symptoms indicative of strongly repressed affect states. Kolb (1985) describes the following behavioral symptoms as primary indicators of massive repression:

- recurrent aggressive/violent episodes, sometimes involving flashbacks
- chronic amnesia re combat traumas
- absence of affective responses in description of extreme traumatization

Also indicative of repression are:

- repetitive panic attacks (unaffected by therapeutic interventions)
- persistent/recurrent pain complaining behavior

Kolb (1985) notes that in situations where there are suspected atrocities that are under repression, it is unwise to initiate narcosynthesis, despite the presence of other indicators.

The major contraindication for the therapeutic use of narco-synthesis is suspected prepsychotic personality characteristics. Kolb (1985) notes that the major concern about employing narcosynthesis is psychotic regression following abreaction. Narcosynthesis is also contra-indicated when patients have diseases involving (1) cardiorespiratory systems; (2) the liver; and (3) the kidneys. "Narcosynthesis is absolutely contraindicated when the patient has porphyria" (p. 218). The major physiological risk is of respiratory delay and/or paralysis. A thorough physical is recommended.

Procedure

At present Kolb (1985) first assesses the patient's hypnotizability and/or capacity to resolve amnestic dissociation within traditional indi-vidual psychotherapy. If hypnotherapy or an uncovering approach can be effective, narcosynthesis is not initiated. When narcosynthesis is in-dicated, Kolb (1985) effects several changes to standard techniques. These include:

- induction of abreaction by audiotape recordings of combat sounds (this avoids verbal suggestion)
- videotaping of the narcosynthetic session
- patient viewing of the videotape with the patient's psychiatrist or with others

The goal of the procedure is to relieve the inner tension of the patient. Naturally the patient is prepared for the treatment and the required support staff are present.

Effectiveness

Kolb (1985) summarizes the effectiveness of narcosynthesis as follows:

> [F]ollow-up studies suggest narcosynthesis as valuable in attenuating the risk for recurrent dissociative states, which are associated with socially destructive, acting out behavior. Confrontation of the denied and unre-vealed emotionally charged experience from which the dissociative behavior has been derived, through viewing of the audiovisually recorded abreaction, has been useful in initiation of later continuing group therapy, individual therapy, or both (p. 222).

Kolb (1985) adds that the material gleaned from narcosynthesis was frequently missed during other diagnostic procedures. Frequently nar-cosynthesis relieves feelings of inner tension and depression. However, the "constant symptoms" of PTSD are often unaffected.

12

Group Treatment

INTRODUCTION

Although individual treatment of psychological problems has been the characteristic therapeutic response to patients with PTSD, the emergence of the Vietnam combat veterans' self-help movement and "rap groups" (Shatan, 1973) brought focus to the use of group therapy with this population. In many ways the group approach to veterans with PTSD grew out of the rap groups of the 1970s. Walker and Nash (1981) argue that group treatment of Vietnam veterans can be of tremendous benefit to patients who avoid individual treatment out of a feeling that they cannot be understood by the therapist. The presence of other patients with similar experiences and problems is beneficial in reducing resistance. Walker and Nash (1981) also argue that mistrust is also easier to deal with in a group setting, since trust tends to develop relatively naturally between group members.

Despite the fact that the majority of reports on the use of group therapy with PTSD patients is confined to Vietnam veterans, many of the procedures are readily adapted to the treatment of other PTSD patient populations. To the degree that it has been possible, procedures are described without reference to the type of patient with PTSD.

THEORETICAL ORIENTATIONS

Four major theoretical orientations are represented by authors advocating the use of group therapy with patients manifesting PTSD:

(1) interactive; (2) cognitive-behavioral; (3) psychoanalytic; and (4) Jungian. Walker and Nash (1981) and Brende (1981) report on the use of interactively oriented group psychotherapy following the basic psychotherapy principles outlined by Yalom (1975). Although not insight-oriented, they do note that catharsis, support, suggestion, and interaction are characteristic features of their groups. Marafiote (1980) outlines a cognitive-behavioral approach to group therapy with PTSD patients, drawing upon learning theory as a theoretical model of behavior. A psychodynamic orientation has also been advocated. Frick and Bogart (1982) report on the use of a psychoanalytic approach to treating Vietnam veterans with PTSD, with a special focus on transference/countertransference phenomena. Bloch and Bloch (1976) also report on the use of analytic group psychotherapy with "post-traumatic psychoses," although focus on stress-response syndromes appears secondary to a focus on psychotic functioning. Finally, Wilmer (1982a, 1982b) reports on a group Jungian approach that focuses on dreams ("dream seminars"). Although this approach is not specific to patients suffering from PTSD, the groups reported on did include members with PTSD.

PROCEDURES

Interactively Oriented Group Psychotherapy

The procedures for conducting group psychotherapy with Vietnam veterans follow in large part the principles organized by Yalom (1975). From their experience with Vietnam veteran groups, Walker and Nash (1981) make several recommendations:

- Group size should be between 5 and 8 patients.
- Noncombat veterans should not be included in groups with combat veterans.
- A mixture of black and white members is beneficial.
- A cotherapist is advised due to powerful countertransference reactions of the therapists.
- Twice-weekly meetings are preferred.
- Session length should be 1.5 hours.

Walker and Nash (1981) note a number of characteristic difficulties dealt with in veteran groups. These include (1) mistrust; (2) fear of losing control; (3) tenacious character defenses; and (4) guilt. Walker and Nash (1981) recommend various factors under the therapist's direction for appropriately handling the difficulties noted. These include therapist

- empathy, involvement, activity, and consistency
- alignment with the patients and group
- encouragement of interaction
- support of progress in individuals and group
- control during times of intense emotion, especially when violence is feared and painful memories erupt
- maintenance of focus on traumas and ongoing life difficulties
- encouragement of group support for members' confessions

Cognitive-Behavioral Group Treatment

Marafiote (1980) describes a cognitive-behavioral approach to treating Vietnam veterans with PTSD in a group setting. Characteristics of groups included:

- group size: 8–10 veterans
- number of sessions: time-limited, usually 8–12 sessions
- spacing of sessions: biweekly during initial stages; weekly thereafter
- length of sessions: 1.5–2.5 hours

Marafiote (1980) argues that certain general considerations must be attended to in order to facilitate the overall functioning and success of the group. These include:

- the importance of attendance
- making the group experience positively reinforcing
- encouraging comradeship and group cohesiveness (e.g., beginning some sessions early to encourage friendships, instigating a buddy system and telephone exchange, etc.)
- eliciting self-disclosure
- promoting complimentary and supportive statements

Phase I: Orientation and Commitment. Marafiote (1980) recommends an orientation session with one of the therapists for each potential member of the group. The session is used to explain the group functioning to the patient, and also to explore his expectations, interests, and concerns. Most important is the development of a treatment contract, a project continued during the first group session. Marafiote (1980) recommends soliciting and obtaining a written and signed contract of commitment to the group process, arguing that such an act is positively correlated with regular group attendance and improvement.

Phase II: Assessment, Goal Identification/Specification. Once the group has begun meeting regularly, focus shifts to an assessment by the therapist and the group of each member's difficulties. Goal identification/specification follows. This process includes:

- describing difficulties with regard to observable behaviors and cognitions
- defining parameters of behavior (e.g., frequency, intensity, etc.)
- noting antecedents, motoric/verbal-cognitive/physiological components, and consequents for each behavior
- utilizing assessment techniques to gather information (e.g., role-playing and behavioral interview [Cone & Hawkins, 1977; Haynes, 1978; etc.])
- utilizing assessment instruments to collect data (e.g. Life History Questionnaire [Wolpe, 1969]; Rathus Assertiveness Schedule [Rathus, 1973]; Reinforcement Survey Schedule [Homme et al., 1967]; etc.)
- delineating strengths and weaknesses
- setting goals based upon cumulative data (preferably short-term goals)
- defining context, time-frame, criteria for successful completion of goal

Phase III: Techniques and Applications. Marafiote (1980) lists a number of treatment techniques employed in various veteran groups led by a cognitive-behavioral therapist. Clearly, the application of various treatment procedures must be fit to the specific difficulties faced by individual patients. The techniques and applications noted are:

- *Relaxation training* (Bernstein & Borkovec, 1973): several muscle groups may be relaxed at the beginning of a session, relaxation at home encouraged.
- *Thought-stopping* for obsessive/maladaptive thoughts: patient is encouraged to concentrate on anxiety producing thoughts and/or images and then shouts "stop!"; in time, individual takes charge; finally, competing, pleasant thoughts are paired with the "stop!" command.
- *Modeling* (Bandura, 1971) by therapist and other patients.
- *Behavioral rehearsal* plus group feedback; inviting a female therapist to aid in all-male groups can be beneficial.
- *Role playing/reversal:* particularly effective with interactional problems.
- *Assertiveness training,* including out-of-group reading of available books (e.g., Alberti & Emmons, 1978; Fensterheim & Baer, 1975; etc.) by patients.

- *Coverant control:* the use of competing cognitions to interrupt maladaptive cognitive/behavioral patterns, low self-esteem, depression, negative attitude, etc.
- *Cognitive restructuring* (Ellis, 1962; Goldfried & Davidson, 1976).
- *Cognitive rehearsal* (imagination of successful completion of target goal).
- *Contingency contracting* (Rose, 1977; Gelfand & Hartmann, 1975) both within group and outside the group.
- *Homework* (e.g., relaxation, contract, utilizing techniques learned in group) plus record of homework: typically 3 assigned per week.
- *Use of charts and graphs* (e.g., for attendance, homework achievement, etc.).
- *Refunding fees* associated with attendance and completion of homework (e.g., $40 accepted at beginning of treatment, refunded during course of therapy).
- *Personal delivery of bills* (an opportunity for positive reinforcement for hard work in group).
- *Bibliotherapy* (materials selected by therapist for individuals to target certain behaviors).

PSYCHODYNAMICALLY ORIENTED GROUP PSYCHOTHERAPY

Although many authors have argued against the efficacy of psychoanalytic approaches to the treatment of PTSD (e.g., Haley, 1985; Figley, 1978; Fuentes, 1980), Frick and Bogart (1982) contend that a psychoanalytic orientation contributes towards understanding the dynamics within a therapeutic group. Of particular importance are transference/countertransference (T/CT) phenomena. The T/CT in-group processes includes not only the reenactment of childhood patterns, but also those patterns acquired from adult trauma (although they do refer to these transferences as "superficial"). Of particular importance within the Vietnam veteran group treated by Frick and Bogart (1982) was the "unconscious fantasy" that the therapy group was the combat unit in Vietnam.

The group case study presented by Frick and Bogart (1982) describes a single experience with a group of Vietnam veterans. Despite this, many of the ideas are useful and generalizable to other groups comprised of PTSD patients. Characteristics of the group included:

- 6–8 members
- stable, long-term therapy group (not a rap group)
- member homogeneity: all members of the group were combat veterans and suffering from PTSD; all but one were diagnosed as having borderline personality disorders

The phases of treatment described by Frick and Bogart (1982) deal primarily with alterations in the T/CT.

Phase I: Development of Group Cohesion (Sessions 1–10). The initial phase of treatment is described by Frick and Bogart (1982) as one of ventilation and the building of group cohesion. T/CT phenomena included:

- intense anger not directed toward nonveteran therapists
- therapists treated with "mild disdain," often ignored
- questioning of whether therapists could "really understand"
- derivative comments about therapists (discussion of incompetent "green lieutenants" in Vietnam)
- therapist experience of projective identification or complementary CT (Racker, 1957): as inexperienced leaders in Vietnam felt inexperienced, unsure of roles, guilty, etc.
- concordant CT (Racker, 1957) feelings: identification with the veterans' anger and suffering.

Frick and Bogart (1982) report that the ability to distinguish between realistic and unrealistic responses enhanced their ability to be constructive in the group.

Phase II: Catharsis (Approximately Months 2–6). Following the group cohesion established in phase I, the focus of the group became the control of violent and self-destructive impulses. Ground rules were established. Within this structure catharsis came to characterize this stage of group treatment. With respect to T/CT phenomena Frick and Bogart (1982) note:

- increasing anger directed towards therapist
- strong CT responses to reports of atrocities and poor treatment of women, etc.
- other CT responses included: "primitive admiration," awe, envy, vicarious enjoyment of sadism

As with the other group approaches noted earlier, nonjudgmental listening, encouragement of disclosure, the fostering of group support, advancing the grieving process, and the reinforcing of group controls contributed to the resolution of emotional issues.

Phase III: Rage Toward Therapists (Approximately Months 6–8).
T/CT phenomena became particularly intense during phase III. Frick
and Bogart (1982) noted:

- anger at incompetent leaders returned with intensity: directed at
  therapists
- derision of therapists for being in training
- demands face-to-face meeting with supervisors
- suspicion of therapists' motives
- feelings of humiliation associated with previous periods of openness
- interventions ridiculed
- outrage expressed at minor episodes of therapist insensitivity
- CT feelings of "being a prisoner of war"
- CT rage towards patients

To deal with the difficult T/CT dynamics set in motion, Frick and Bogart (1982) admitted mistakes, accepted the group's wrath with as little
defensiveness as possible, contained intense anger/anxiety, admitted
anger when appropriate, and monitored their desires to withdraw from
the group.

*Phase IV: Facing Current Realities (Approximately Months 8–
Termination).* Frick and Bogart (1982) report that following phase III
confrontation between group members became possible. In Kleinian
terms the group shifted from a paranoid-schizoid position to a depressive position (Klein, 1957). Focus turned to depressive feelings and current difficulties. T/CT phenomena at this stage included:

- an idealizing T toward therapists (they had proven themselves
  "under fire")
- CT feelings of elation in response to idealizing T
- CT feelings that the patients were "splitting" (and fear of again
  being attacked, devalued)
- CT feelings that no progress had been made
- upon announcement of termination patients reported feeling rejected, abandoned
- CT feelings of having survived a "tour of duty"

In sum, Frick and Bogart (1982) argue that the psychoanalytically oriented approach to group treatment facilitated revivification and the
working through of traumatic memories. Further, they describe the
group as a "transitional culture" for the veterans as they sought to be
reintegrated into the society at large.

DREAM SEMINARS

Wilmer (1982a, 1982b) describes the development of "dream seminars" for inpatients in a V.A. hospital. As noted earlier, although all members of the dream seminar groups were veterans, only a proportion of those participating were suffering specifically from PTSD. However, PTSD patients are focused upon in case examples. Wilmer (1982a) argues that the dreams of Vietnam veterans contain "an unconscious history of the war." He notes the tremendous relief of veterans when their dreams were attended to and taken seriously. Wilmer (1982a) also noted the mixture of personal and archetypal contents to the veterans dreams. Out of these experiences the dreams seminars were developed.

Characteristics of dreams seminars include (Wilmer 1982a, 1982b):

- seminar led by therapist experienced with dreamwork
- focus on so-called "manifest" level of the dream
- an emphasis on learning and teaching
- inclusion of all patients (including chronic schizophrenics)
- patients sit in a circle
- when patient population greater than 20, two concentric circles formed
- once a week meetings
- length of meetings one hour

Wilmer (1982b) notes that working with dreams does not aggravate conditions such as psychosis. The procedures for working within the group include (Wilmer, 1982a, 1982b):

- Statement by therapist (each session) of what the dream seminar was (e.g., working with dreams can help patient tend to difficulties and promote healing).
- Therapist asks for a patient to share a dream (preferably from previous night).
- Therapist repeats dream to the group.
- Patients ask dreamer to clarify images and story of dream (focus on dream images, not on interpretation).
- Dreamer asked what is happening in his life (about which the dream may be commenting).
- Group members offer comment ("interpretation").
- Therapist sums up ("interpretation").
- At times parts of a dream may be reenacted (gestalt-like psychodrama directed by therapist).
- Focus on one, possibly two, dreams in an hour.
- With more than 20 patients attending, only the inner circle works, the outer circle watches; later the circles change places.

Wilmer (1982a) argues that when the unconscious dream material of Vietnam veterans is attended to, as in dream seminars, acceptance and reintegration of the traumatic experience is facilitated. "The Dream Seminar offers a worthwhile balance to the one-sidedness of many therapies which automatically and rigidly exclude unconscious and preconscious processes" (Wilmer, 1982b, p. 359). In particular he notes that insomnia is often reduced. Indeed, on the unit described by Wilmer (1982a, 1982b) sleeping medications were not routinely prescribed; instead patients were encouraged to talk to nurses and to work with dreams they might have had (e.g., tell them to the nurses, paint the dream images, or save them until the next dream seminar). Wilmer (1982a) argues that attention to the dreams of Vietnam veterans promotes the understanding and integration of the "collective shadow" which has been projected onto soldiers of the Vietnam conflict. Wilmer (1982a, 1982b) notes that dream seminar work is welcomed by patients (i.e, the dream seminars were the only group function punctually attended by patients).

COMBINED INDIVIDUAL AND GROUP THERAPY

Brende (1981) has argued in favor of combined individual and group therapy for Vietnam veterans. He argues that

- trust cannot be developed solely in the context of group therapy
- individual plus group therapy enhances revivification
- individual therapist brings additional support to patient
- different information is revealed, and different experiences obtained, from individual and group therapy—both are beneficial

Brende (1981) notes that some patients have difficulty discussing their war traumas in individual therapy, and thus group therapy can further treatment in that area. Group also enhances socialization and the dissolving of mistrust, factors attended to less by individual treatment approaches. From the other direction, some patients so overidentify with the other members in the group that individual therapy is beneficial for them.

EFFECTIVENESS

The effectiveness of group therapy with PTSD patients has only been described anecdotally in the literature. However, given the reported efficacy of rap groups for Vietnam veterans (Shatan, 1973), as well as the reports of efficacy reported by Walker and Nash (1981), Brende (1981), Marafiote (1980), Frick and Bogart (1982), and Wilmer (1982a, 1982b) group therapy would appear to be a viable treatment approach for treating PTSD patients.

13

Family and Couples Therapy

INTRODUCTION

As noted earlier, stress-response syndromes have been resisted by the mental health community until relatively recently. Indeed, it is still the cause of debate between various theoretical positions. As Figley and Sprenkle (1978) and Schultz (1984) stress, the families of PTSD patients have also been largely ignored. Consequently, as Scurfield (1985) states, little attention has been given to the impact of PTSD on families and family treatment of families with a member suffering from PTSD.

The majority of approaches to patients with PTSD have focused upon the individual. Given the impairment in interpersonal functioning commonly found with PTSD patients, Figley and Sprenkle (1978) argue that the family and the family therapist are in a unique position to help PTSD patients. Stanton and Figley (1978) assert that family therapy has the potential of eliminating PTSD in the family member experiencing the disorder. Also, since the children of families with a parent suffering from PTSD are often adversely affected, for example children of holocaust survivors (Danieli, 1985), family therapy can be beneficial to more than just the PTSD patient.

As with the majority of the literature dealing with PTSD, papers on family therapy and PTSD are focused primarily on Vietnam veteran families. However, many of the characteristics found in such families, and many of the concepts reported for dealing with problems, can directly inform family therapy with other PTSD patient populations. An exception to the trend of reports on family therapy with Vietnam Veterans, is the work by Danieli (1985) on holocaust families

THEORETICAL ASSUMPTIONS

The overarching theoretical positions adopted by family therapists dealing with PTSD patients and their families are that of a systems (or interpersonal) orientation (Bertalanffy, 1968; Figley, 1988) and a cybernetics orientation (Maruyama, 1963). Although various authors utilize different specific concepts from within family therapy, all agree that the PTSD patient both affects the family and is, in turn, affected by the family. Thus the interaction of the patient with those around him/her, as well as the difficulties the patient is having intrapsychically, is the focus of therapy. The primary unit of treatment is the family.

PROCEDURES

The specific therapeutic procedures utilized by family therapists treating families of PTSD patients depends largely upon their orientation. A review of the literature dealing with family therapy for PTSD conditions reveals therapists using, among others, the theoretical frameworks and techniques of Alexander and Parsons (1981), Bowen (1976, 1978), Haley (1976), Minuchin (1974), Satir (1972), and Weakland et al. (1974).

Given the fact that family problems may extend beyond the immediate difficulties in integrating the post-traumatic experience into the family system, no standard course of treatment can be predicted (Figley & Spenkle, 1978; Figley, 1988). However, the presence of a member of the family with PTSD does introduce certain qualities of treatment which must be specifically addressed.

GOALS OF FAMILY THERAPY

Figley (1988) has delineated four goals of family treatment. The first goal is rapport building and clarifying the therapist's role. In addition, the roles of the family as members of the therapeutic procedure are also clarified. The following parameters are generally applicable:

> (1) in most cases the actual therapy will be relatively brief, (2) the role of the therapist is to *facilitate* (original italics) recovery and self-reliance, (3) the task

of the family is to refine and develop their own skills for coping with extraordinary circumstance, (4) success will not only improve current circumstances, but enable the family to cope more successfully with future ordeals,
and (5) they can—individually and as a family—be useful to others attempting to cope with similar circumstances. (Figley, 1988, p. 96)

The second goal is the development of new rules and skills of family
communication (Figley, 1988). The frame of reference that therapists
want to create with these families is that the purpose of therapy is to
"facilitate effective coping with extraordinary events, those in which the
family has very little experience...[and coping] with extraordinary circumstances, requires extraordinary methods (rules and communication
skills)" (Figley, 1988, p. 97). The family can decide whether these new
behaviors can be viewed as temporary changes to cope with the trauma
or permanent changes.

For some families the rules of communication as well as the roles of
family members may have been dysfunctional or only marginally functional before the trauma. In other families, these parameters of the
system may have been adaptive prior to the trauma, but insufficiently
flexible to accommodate to the new environmental demands. In still
other situations, the trauma may have been so devastating that almost
any family would not be able to adjust without help. Therapists may
want to pay attention to these diagnostic considerations in order to have
some "appropriate expectation" about the family flexibility. However,
from a strategic standpoint, these considerations may not matter a great
deal if the family is induced into the framework of extraordinary problems need extraordinary solutions.

The third goal is self-disclosure. The fourth goal is recapitulation
of the traumatic events (Figley, 1988). The essential principle in these
aspects of therapy is the cessation of avoidant behavior in all parts of the
family. As each person is allowed and encouraged to describe his or her
individual reactions to the trauma and the effects of the trauma on
other family members (Figley, 1988), increased differentiation can occur. In addition, family members have the opportunity to feel a greater
sense of intimacy with other members. Individuals often have similar or
parallel experiences of pain and suffering. Yet, they bare their feelings
all alone. Gradually, individuals in the family discover that part of the
"healing" is derived not from getting rid of the pain; it is a function of
sharing the pain with loved ones. Furthermore, since there is a greater
sharing of information, more varied points of view and possible solutions are generated.

The final goal is the building of a "family healing theory." Figley
(1988) follows Horowitz's (1986) work about the importance of developing new realities about the causes of the event. We would add that the

works of Epstein (1990) and Janoff-Bulman (1985) are also relevant. The family is literally to come up with a single theory of what happened, why each person acted as they did (both during and following the event), and lastly, with an optimistic image of how the family should react should a similar event occur again.

CHARACTERISTICS OF POST-TRAUMATIC FAMILIES

Families of Vietnam veterans with PTSD are characterized by a variety of common features and recurring interactionally based patterns (Figley & Sprenkle, 1978; Stanton & Figley, 1978; Goodwin, 1980; Jurich, 1983; Marrs, 1985; Schultz, 1984; Williams & Williams, 1985). It is important these be assessed. These include, with respect to the PTSD patient:

- veterans viewed as "identified patients"
- substance abuse
- outbursts of violence and rage by veteran
- "identity foreclosure" in PTSD patient
- poor veteran self-concept due to current inability to control impulses and failure to fulfill role as husband/father
- lack of ability of veteran to empathize with illness and loss
- emotional isolation/alienation of veteran from spouse and children

Problems experienced by wives of veterans include:

- abuse (emotional, verbal, and physical)
- neglecting their own emotional needs due to focus on "crisis-responding"
- frequently feeling guilty that the problems are entirely their fault;
- frequently becoming primary financial/emotional support of the family and feeling overwhelmed
- depression and low self-esteem in women partners
- feeling frustrated in their ability to help

Problems experienced between partners include:

- violent episodes perpetuated by both partners
- problems with intimacy in both partners
- unfaithfulness by veterans
- "disengaged" dyadic patterns
- functional female partner/dysfunctional male partner pattern

Children can develop a wide range of behavioral symptoms. PTSD patients can turn to their children, rather than their spouses, for nurturance and intimacy.

Problems characteristic of the entire family system include:

- rigid patterns of family interaction
- unspoken rules (e.g., Vietnam traumas will not be discussed)
- tendency for family to "aggravate" the patient's problems (e.g., rigid reinforcement of denial/numbing, inciting patient to act out, etc.)
- reaction of family system to PTSD symptomatology
- isolation from extended family, friends, community, etc.

Recently, Danieli (1985) has outlined characteristics common among holocaust survivor families. These findings were based on work with 75 survivors of the holocaust and 300 children of survivors. Four types of families are conceptualized: "victim families," "fighter families," "numb families," and "families of those who made it." Within victim families the following characteristics were noted:

- home atmosphere marked by depression, worry, mistrust, fear of outside world
- mistrust instilled in children
- overreactions to everyday events
- symbiotic clinging within family
- separation feared by parents and children
- independence discouraged
- marked overinvolvement and overprotectiveness of children
- frequent marital/sexual difficulties in children's families
- fear of having children among children
- somatization used to control family members
- an emphasis on "being right" and "in control"
- children pulled into marital difficulties
- guilt used to control family members
- fear among children of surpassing their parents with concomitant destruction of their own success

Within "fighter families" Danieli (1985) noted:

- intense/compulsive drive to build/achieve
- weakness/self-pity not permitted
- illness equals narcissistic insult
- mistrust of outside authorities; aggression against outsiders

Within "numb families" Danieli (1985) noted:

- pervasive silence in home

- "depletion of all emotions"
- tolerance of only a minimal amount of stimulation
- spontaneity/fantasy in children impaired
- children often adopt outsiders as "family" as compensation
- children feel unattended to, unimportant

The characteristics of "families who made it" include (Danieli, 1985):

- active and powerful desire for higher education, social/political status, fame, wealth, etc.
- "normal"/acculturated posture assumed
- denial/avoidance of past with concomitant numbing, isolation, somatization
- high rates of divorce
- survivor center of family; children report feeling neglected

In addition to an assessment of the various problems listed above, Stanton and Figley (1978) recommend an assessment of various issues with respect to the family of origin (FOO) and family of procreation (FOP). The family of origin refers to the patient's parents and siblings. The family of procreation refers to the patient's spouse and children. With respect to the FOO they suggest inquiring about:

- differentiation from FOO by PTSD patient
- recent events in FOO (e.g., deaths and divorces)
- reactions by PTSD patient of events in FOO
- possible systemic purposes of any handicap in PTSD patient
- issues of anger/violence related to FOO

With respect to FOP:

- length of marital relationship
- any changes that have taken place in the course of the marriage
- stresses on the family (e.g., financial and social)
- the possibility PTSD symptoms obscure deeper problems
- the possibility that were the PTSD patient to recover his/her spouse would leave

Although the above lists have been drawn from the literature on Vietnam veteran families and holocaust survivor families, many of these characteristics are also typical of family reactions to patients with PTSD derived from another stressor.

PHASES OF TREATMENT

Figley (1988) and Jurich (1983) have both described different phases of treatment with families. In his work with families of Vietnam veterans, Jurich (1983) describes (1) pre-treatment; (2) intake/assessment; (3) ventilation; (4) bridging; (5) education; and (6) taking the therapy home. In describing his work with unspecified types of post-traumatic problems, Figley (1988) delineates five phases to therapy: (1) building commitment to the therapeutic objectives; (2) framing the problem; (3) reframing the problem; (4) developing a healing theory; and (5) closure and preparedness. Jurich (1983) and Figley (1988) use different labels for defining the first three phases of therapy. However, they are describing essentially the same process. These phases will be described in synthetic format. The remaining phases do not lend themselves for synthesis, so they will be examined separately.

Phase 1: Assessment and Building Rapport. The first differential issue that confronts the therapist is whether or not the family defines the problem as a trauma-related disorder. If the family does label the problem as trauma-related, then clinicians can make their assessments (as described in Chapter 6). Figley (1988) and McCubbin & Figley (1983) have described several other family parameters that merit evaluation. Questions to be answered include: Is a clear stressor defined? Does the family blame one individual or do they see the problem as a family problem? Other issues include: the presence of violence, the presence of drugs and alcohol, family role flexibility, and amount of affection between family members (Figley, 1988; McCubbin & Figley, 1983).

Following the work of the MRI school of family therapy (Weakland et al., 1974), Figley and Sprenkle (1978) point out that many times the family's attempt to solve the problem actually aggravates it. In particular, Figley and Sprenkle (1978) cite the tendency of some families of Vietnam veterans to reinforce the denial and numbing tendencies of the PTSD victims. In these families, the message is sent not to talk about the problem, get on with business, and so on. Other families reinforce the intrusive phase of the disorder. These families can be more dangerous. If the trauma victim tends to act out rage, and the response of the family is also inflammatory, then violence can escalate.

Often the family does not label the problem as trauma-related. Jurich (1983) notes that, for families of Vietnam veterans with PTSD, the initial complaint is generally adolescent rebellion. Goodwin (1980) comments that family violence often brings the family in for treatment. War-related trauma is often not mentioned, and would be resisted if the topic were brought up directly (Jurich, 1983).

One way clinicians can get an approximation of the degree of trauma-related dysfunction is to ask general questions about the different stresses that family members have had. Has anyone been in the armed service? Has anyone been the victim of a violent act?—and so on. If the family is overly defended, then it would prudent not to jump on the trauma issue immediately. Jurich (1983) described a technique termed "age-sounding" where a family member who is quite upset is asked how old he or she feels. Once the age is defined then the problems of that age are discussed. Usually, it is the age that the person was experiencing some type of trauma.

Ideally, the family will identify the trauma as a relevant issue for the family early in treatment. Figley (1988) emphasizes the following goals in the initial stage of treatment: (1) the disclosure of the ordeal by the family members; (2) delineation of specific treatment objectives; (3) the therapist conveying a high degree of confidence; and (4) the therapist projecting a sense of optimism for a positive treatment outcome.

Phase II: Ventilation and Framing the Problem. The second phase of therapy involves the family members discussing the trauma. The successful conclusion of this phase of therapy results in self-disclosure among the family (Figley, 1988), the "family myth" about not being able to talk about the trauma being disconfirmed (Jurich, 1983), and attention is shifted away from the "victim" toward the entire family system (Figley, 1988; Jurich, 1983).

Jurich (1983) terms this phase "ventilation;" Figley (1988) terms it "framing the problem." Therapeutic strategies for this phase include (1) allowing family members to articulate their own views and reactions to the relevant traumatic event; (2) promoting recognition and acceptance of the meaningfulness of each family member's personal experience (this is a special case of promoting differentiation); and (3) allowing the family to list both the undesirable and desirable consequences of the trauma (Figley, 1988).

One other type of information is important to acquire in this phase of the treatment. Both therapist and family members need to review what the attempts at problem solution have been up to the present. Not only will this let the clinician know how the attempts at problem resolution have aggravated the situation (Figley & Sprenkle, 1978), it will provide information for the next phase of therapy.

Phase III: Reframing the Problem. Figley (1988) states that this phase is the most critical one of the therapy. The goal involves "bridging" the differences between family members within the system (Jurich, 1983). Each family member will have their own individual set of assumptions (Janoff-Bulman, 1985) and personal theories about their motivations and the motivations of others (Epstein, 1989). To varying extents these theories about what happened and why it happened will be shared by other family members. The therapist must help reframe the different experiences of the family members so that they will be compatible with the final construction of the healing theory (Figley, 1988). Jurich (1983) has delineated a number of techniques to achieve these goals. They are (1) normalizing behavior; (2) relabeling behavior; (3) positively connotating behavior; (4) redefining family patterns; (5) facilitating recognition of similarities among family members; and (6) facilitating the discovery of "new meaning" within the family.

Phase IV: Developing a Healing Theory. Figley (1988) emphasizes that unlike an individual healing theory (that might be the result of therapy along the lines set down by Epstein (1989), Horowitz (1986) or Janoff-Bullman (1985)), the family healing theory must be embraced by *all of the family members.* The theory will be generated from statements that are made during the previous therapy sessions. The statements may have been made spontaneously or as a result of accepting reframing interventions.

Jurich (1983) discusses two other phases of treatment. These are "education" and "taking the therapy home." The former revolves around communication skills training. Jurich (1983) advocates a paradoxical stance of stressing that the family not try their newly learned skills at home for a while. The hope is that this will prevent the unstructured home environment from undermining therapeutic advances. Of course, the family can "resist" and prove the therapist wrong by successfully practicing the new skills at home. The latter phase calls for using the new skills at home. It is started once the family has consolidated its gains.

While these phases are not at odds with Figley's (1988) work, they appear to be more germane to the structural difficulties of any family. The development of a healing theory would be more specific to a traumatized family.

TREATMENT STRATEGIES/GOALS

The goal of family treatment with PTSD patients includes (Figley & Sprenkle, 1978; Jurich, 1983):

- a safe and supportive family environment in which feelings and thoughts associated with the traumatic experience can be shared and discussed
- restructure of the family so that all members are age-appropriately differentiated

• generalization of skills/learning to home environment

Williams and Williams (1985) suggest focus on the following issues for helping impaired families achieve these characteristics:

• removal of veteran from identified patient role
• providing alternate strategies for coping with rage/violence
• enhancing discussion/integration of traumatic experiences into family system
• education about characteristics of PTSD (e.g., the veteran/family is not "crazy")
• promoting mutual support by partners
• skills training (e.g., communication exercises, assertiveness training, conflict-resolution, parenting skills, coping with stress, etc.)
• differentiation from culturally stereotyped roles
• clarification of values

The majority of these focal points would appear best addressed in phases III and IV of treatment.

THE THERAPIST'S ROLE

The therapist attempting to help the PTSD patient faces a variety of problems, not the least of which is the patient's sense that the therapist does not "really understand" the traumatic experience. To facilitate the feeling on the part of the patient that he/she is understood, Figley and Sprenkle (1978) have suggested cotherapy wherein one of the therapists is himself or herself a recovered PTSD patient (e.g., a currently functioning combat veteran, rape victim, disaster survivor, etc.). This is particularly important when the patient comes to a point in therapy where the original trauma becomes the focus of treatment.

In addition to introducing the changes and procedures noted earlier, the role of the therapist includes (Figley & Sprenkle, 1978) (1) modeling appropriate behavior; (2) facilitating role rehearsal; (3) deciding when to include/exclude children; and (4) deciding when individual sessions may be appropriate deciding when physical separations of family members may be appropriate (e.g., due to violence).

INTEGRATION OF FAMILY THERAPY
WITH OTHER MODALITIES

Williams and Williams (1985) note that family therapy can be used as an adjct to, or in conjuction, with a variety of other treatment modalities. These include (1) individual therapy/counseling; (2) veteran group therapy; (3) marital/couples therapy; (4) multiple couples groups; (5) community education and outreach; (6) individual therapy/counseling for partner of veteran; (7) women partners groups; and (8) substance abuse treatment (in-/outpatient)

PROBLEMATIC PERIODS

Family therapy with families of PTSD patients will likely be affected by transitional points in the patient's life (Erikson, 1968) and major transitions in the family life cycle (Stanton & Figley, 1978).

EFFECTIVENESS

To date, the effectiveness of family therapy for treating families with a member manifesting PTSD has not been addressed at large. The exception to this is a case report by Schultz (1984) in which strategic therapy techniques were successful improving a Vietnam veteran's adjustment difficulties.

14

Therapy of Children with PTSD

INTRODUCTION

Unfortunately, there has been little published material on the therapy of children who have experienced trauma or disaster. Generally, there are three types of specialized interventions that have been described: Individual Psychodynamic (Pynoos & Eth, 1986), Group Play Therapy (Galante & Foa, 1986) and Group Stress Inoculation Training (Ayalon, 1983). It is not clear how the majority of children who experience trauma receive treatment. Presumably, they are either treated in family therapy (see Chapter 13) or general individual play therapy (usually psychodynamic in nature).

Pynoos & Eth (1986) describe in great detail a 90-minute interview format that they have used with over 200 children who have witnessed severe violence (e.g., murder, rape, suicide, kidnapping, school or community violence). The interview is designed for children 3–16 years of age who *recently* experienced trauma. Before the interview itself clinicians should have information from outside sources (e.g., family or police) about the event, the family circumstance, and the child's reaction to the trauma. In this way the interviewers can be aware of important references or omissions during the session.

STAGE 1: OPENING

Establishing a Focus. Once the child is greeted, a focus for the session is set by telling that the clinician has had experience in talking to children who have "gone through what you have gone through" (p. 307). An alternative is to say that you are interested in understanding what that child has gone through.

Free Drawing and Storytelling. The child is asked to draw whatever he or she likes and to tell a story about it. It is emphasized that by leaving the child to draw alone, the child is more likely to apply himself to the drawing. The child can be asked to elaborate on the drawing or the story by wondering about a detail or asking what happens next.

Traumatic Reference. The clinician must find the reference to the traumatic event that is inevitably present in the drawing and or the story.

STAGE 2: TRAUMA

Emotional Release. Once the reference to trauma is discerned the therapist needs carefully to open the wound by linking reference in the story or drawing to the trauma. For example: (1) "Your father could have been saved like the clown;" or (2) "Your baby-sitter could have gotten away from the man who was about to stab her" (p. 308).

In the first example the child had drawn a net underneath a falling clown. The second child made a reference to Bugs Bunny outrunning his attacker. The authors point out that at this point:

> What often follows is a profound emotional outcry from the child. Now the child needs to feel the interviewer's willingness to be a supportive presence and to protect the child from being overwhelmed by the intensity or pro-longation of the emotional release. (p. 308).

Reconstruction. The next segment of the interview is designed to help the child put words to the experience. The authors describe a process whereby the child is led to talk about, enact, and/or draw each aspect of the experience. The direction of the interview is from the more general to the more specific and the more traumatic. It is stressed that the child must experience a sense of safety and hope that he or she will survive talking about the experience. The role of the interviewer is to provide a holding environment that on the one hand allows the child to be safe. On the other hand, the interviewer insures that the child is not allowed to digress from the task. Of course, sensitivity to the child's level of physical and emotional exhaustion is important. Rest, relaxation, and snacks should be offered to allow the child to recoup and to feel cared for during the ordeal of the session. After the snack, the child is focused on the next step in the process.

The child is taken through the following aspects of the trauma:

- The central action the child witnessed when physical harm was inflicted.
- *The perceptual experience of the child.* The sights, sounds, and smells of which the child was aware. It is also important to ask the child about his or her kinesthetic experience.
- *The worst moment.* Once the child has survived the above accounts, which generally have led to increased mastery, the child can be asked about the worst moment. It may be something quite different from what the adult may have expected. The authors note that this point of the interview is one where the child feels particularly understood and close to the interviewer.

COPING WITH THE TRAUMATIC EXPERIENCE

Issues of Human Accountability. The child needs to face the awareness and conflicts over who is to blame. The child can be asked, "How come it happened?" And then, "What would make someone do something like that?"

Inner Plans of Action. These are fantasies about actions that would have remedied the situation. Their character will be in accord with the child's developmental age. In any event, the child needs to be allowed to verbalize or enact these wishes. Young children may choose to flee. School-age children tend to turn passive outlooks into more active perspectives. They can imagine calling the police or locking the doors or taking the weapon away from the assailant.

Punishment and Retaliation. The child is allowed to give full expression to feelings of revenge and punishment. They can be asked, "What would you like to see happen to him?" The child can be helped to feel comfortable with these feelings by saying, "I see it feels good to imagine getting back at the bad man who stabbed your father." Reality can be introduced by adding, " I mean, to be able to do something to him now, when you really could not have stopped him at the time."

Counter-Retaliation. The child may be afraid that the assailant will return. The child needs to be reassured about these issues.

Child's Impulse Control. If the child attributes the violence to actions based on poor control of emotions (e.g., anger or rejection), the child can be asked, "What do you do when you get angry?" The child has witnessed adults' lack of control and may also fear his or her capacity to control feelings.

Traumatic Dreams and Previous Trauma. These are relevant questions that should be asked at this point.

Future Orientation. It is important to ask about the child's concerns about the future.

Current Stresses. The child can be asked about current stresses. It is especially important to discover if there have been important oversights in the child's care since the trauma. The authors state that they offer to help the child fix any of these problems.

STAGE 3: CLOSURE

Recapitulation. The session is reviewed and summarized. This process can be started by returning to the child's first drawing. The child's responses are framed as understandable, realistic and common reactions to such traumatic experiences.

Realistic fears. The child is reminded that his or her emotional responses were normal. It was all right to be scared, and then angry, and so on. If the child has not expressed reasonable fears over his own safety, the interviewer can empathize with how scary it must have been.

Expectable Course. The child is told about the common reactions that often happen. These include feeling scared all of a sudden, thinking about the lost loved one, startle reactions, bad dreams, and so on. It is suggested that the child tell a trusted adult about these reactions.

Child's Courage. The child's self-esteem needs support. The child can be complimented on his or her courage to talk about these difficult issues. Pynoos and Eth report that children always swell with pride upon hearing the words "You were very brave."

Child's Critique. The child is asked to describe what has been most helpful or disturbing about the interview. Usually, children will speak quite openly.

Leavetaking. It is useful to express to the child the interviewer's respect for the child and thanking the child for the privilege of having been able to share the experience with him or her. The child should be given the interviewer's professional card. It is important that the child knows that the opportunity for future contact exists.

In discussing this interview technique Pynoos and Eth (1986) offer the following elaborations. They emphasize that children often report that the discussion or picture drawing about the child's revenge fantasies helped them most. Behaviorally, a perceivable increase of spontaneity is often noticed after this stage. When this step was not successful, continued affective constriction was noted. The final phase of the interview needs to be complete. Insufficient closure can undermine the entire interview. The authors point out that despite some people's fears that this type of interview will further traumatize the children, in fact it brings immediate relief.

The authors point out that there is considerable similarity between their technique and the ones used for the treatment of soldiers who have seen a buddy killed or maimed in action.

Pynoos and Eth (1986) anecdotally state that children improve after this single interview. It is unfortunate that there are not any hard data, such as before-and-after measures. The authors point out that they are guarded about the long-term benefits of a single session. They describe their hope that the single session will help prevent constriction in children . It is hoped that the ability of children to communicate with an adult, which was nurtured in the interview, will be transferred to other caretakers.

Galante and Foa (1986) described a study of 300 Italian elementary school children who were victims of a devastating earthquake. There were six different villages studied. Children were evaluated 6 months post-earthquake.[22] Treatment was offered to the village with the most children at risk. Then the children were evaluated again 18 months post-quake. Sixty-two children, in the first through fourth grades, received treatment. The children who had received the treatment showed a significant drop in at risk scores.

The treatment consisted of seven 1-hour group therapy sessions with four children in each group. There was one session approximately every 4–6 weeks. Each session had a particular theme or objective: Furthermore, the children's behavior changed in correspondence with the different themes of the session.

We have already discussed the work of Ayalon (1983) in the behavior therapy section. The stages of treatment were (1) ventilation of feelings (using verbal and nonverbal modalities); (2) abreaction through

Table 14.1. Group Play Therapy of Children: Objectives, Activities, Responses[a]

Session objective	Session activity	Children's response
Session 1: Give permission to communicate openly about earthquake.	Drawing while listening to stories about San Francisco's recovery from earthquakes and its seismic proof constructions	The children were either aggressive with each other or silent and apprehensive. Nevertheless, they were attentive to the story. Their drawings depicted dangerous environments, full of menacing features.
Session 2: To openly discuss fears, and to demonstrate that being afraid was a common shared reaction.	Drawing while listening to a story about a child who is afraid, but too timid to ask for help. Discussion about their drawings and feelings.	Many children talked about the earthquakes. There were many fears of impending doom.
Session 3: Discuss myths and erroneous beliefs about earthquakes.	Drawing while listening to a story about a child being afraid of earthquakes recurring because he did not understand how they occurred. Discussion about the children's beliefs. A lesson on earthquakes.	A sharp increase in expression of fears and retelling of earthquake stories.
Session 4: Involve children in active discharge of feelings about the earthquake, and place the earthquake in the past.	Making a large joint drawing of the village, furnishing it with small toys. Focus was centered on what was done after the quake to resume normal life.	Increase in exaggerated ways of behaving and displays of emotion. Drawings (in addition to the group project) began to have symbolic reference to actual losses.
Session 5: Release the power of the images of the deaths and focus on building the future.	Role playing and funeral rituals. The future of the new village was planned.	Children played earthquake games. There was an attempt to put order on the disaster. The trauma was framed into a more manageable frame. There was strong and possessive attachment to the investigator. Open references to actual losses were drawn on the pictures.
Session 6: Develop the idea that one is not a "victim of the fate" but could take an active part in one's own survival.	Role-playing being parents teaching children to survive in various emergency situations.	Decrease in intensity of previous session. Role-playing in a more relaxed fashion. Almost no talk of fear despite role-playing of disaster scenes. "Children planned for the future with some skepticism." Doubts were related to realistic concerns.
Session 7: Give the children an opportunity to bring up whatever they chose to in closing.	Free drawing and discussion	Children talked and made pictures about everyday events. They did not discuss earthquake-related themes.

[a]From Galante and Foa (1986).

role-play and retelling of the events; (3) aggression channeling through the use of puppets and plays (the execution of the terrorists brought relief); (4) gradual *in vivo* exposure. (Gradual exposure to noises was carried out, using systematic desensitization procedures. Parents took the children to the beach where the terrorists landed. The *in vivo* exposure was deemed most effective.); (5) cognitive reappraisal of the experience by looking at their behaviors and reactions in light of retrospective knowledge; (6) working through (characterized by more structured activities such as writing poems and erecting memorials); (7) mapping alternatives (which involve making suggestions for future encounters with danger based on all the current information).

Ayalon reports that the group therapy was based on principles of stress inoculation training. Nevertheless, all of the treatments bear striking similarities to the other interventions, that far outweigh their differences.

Stages 1–3 of Ayalon's program are similar to those described by both Pynoos and Eth (1986) and Galante and Foa (1986). Ayalon (1983) and Pynoos and Eth (1986) place considerable importance on the child expressing revenge fantasies. However, it should be pointed out that Galante and Foa (1986) were working with a natural disaster. The other authors were working with human violence.

All of the treatments emphasize the importance of preventing the child from using avoidance. Ayalon's (1983) Stage 4 is carried out *in vivo*, whereas the other authors use *in vitro* methods. Pynoos and Eth (1986) focus specifically on the affective part of the experience.

All of the authors report interventions in the child's appraisal system of what they could have done. Ayalon (1983) appears to be the most specific about this goal. Galante and Foa's (1986) had similar objectives in their therapy. Similarly, Pynoos and Eth (1986) discuss the child's "inner plans of action."

Ayalon (1983) and Galante and Foa (1986) encourage the symbolic working through of the grief through the use of rituals and structured activity. This is one step that is not at all described in the more psychodynamic focus of Pynoos and Eth (1986). However, it should be mentioned that their work tends to occur much closer to the crisis. It would probably be premature to attempt to put closure on the children's grief so early.

All of the authors discuss some type of intervention for helping the child deal with the future stress. Each treatment had a slightly different emphasis.

There are several differences in emphasis worth mentioning. Most important is Pynoos and Eth's (1986) emphasis on strengthening the child's self esteem through discussing the child's courage. It is probable that in practice the other treatments included such interventions. Pynoos and Eth (1986) also raised the issue of counter-retaliation fantasies. This may be specifically relevant in cases of individual crime (There is some reality to this fear, as well as pseudo-reality in the guise of movies and TV where the bad guy comes back). The detailed telling of the trauma discussed by Pynoos and Eth (1986) is also an important difference from the other approaches.

SUMMARY

The three types of interventions described in this chapter conform to all of the common factors in the treatment of PTSD described in Chapter 7. Therefore, we must conclude that the goals of therapy with children suffering from PTSD are essentially equivalent to the goals of working with adults. Obviously, the medium of the therapy needs to be geared to the child (e.g., using pictures and enactment). In the best of all worlds, it would probably be useful to combine the best of all three approaches.

One might expect that it would be best to start with an individual session such as the one described by Pynoos and Eth (1986). Then, the child could be placed in a group treatment. Common to each of these procedures is to help the child examine, confront, and master the stressful experience and accompanying feelings. A number of child-related activities (e.g., picture-drawing, puppet-play, story-telling, and fantasy play) have been used.

15

Psychopharmacological Treatment

INTRODUCTION

Psychopharmacological treatment of PTSD often occurs in conjunction with psychotherapeutic approaches. In his review, van der Kolk (1988) found that there have been clinical reports claiming success for every class of psychoactive medication for specific features of PTSD, including monamine oxidase inhibitors (MAOI), benzodiazepines, tricyclic antidepressants, lithium carbonate, beta-adrenergic blockers, and clonidine. Nevertheless, there have yet to be any controlled studies on any of these compounds (Friedman, 1988; van der Kolk, 1988). At the present time, psychopharmacological treatment of PTSD alone is never sufficient to alleviate the suffering associated with the disorder (Friedman, 1988).

RATIONALES FOR DRUG THERAPY

There are several rationales for adding a psychopharmacological intervention to psychotherapy (whichever form is used). The first rationale is essentially utilitarian. In some cases, the intensity of the symptoms (e.g., anxiety, depression, sleep disturbances, autonomic arousal, and intrusive thoughts) is so great that the symptoms prevent adaptive coping. It is postulated that the reduction of these symptoms through medication prevents additional traumatization (Roth, 1988). Additionally, if painful symptoms are kept within reasonable limits, psychotherapeutic work can be facilitated (Friedman, 1988).

The second rationale is more theoretical. To the extent that PTSD is deemed a biologically driven disorder, it would be logical to utilize medications that influence the biological systems that are postulated as responsible for the disorder (van der Kolk, 1988). The symptoms most associated with PTSD (i.e., intrusive thoughts and hyperarousal) are the ones that have most evidence for a biological basis (van der Kolk et al., 1984, 1985). They are also the same symptoms most successfully treated with medication (Friedman, 1988; van der Kolk, 1988). Avoidant symptoms (e.g., alienation and psychic numbing) rarely respond to medication unless they are the result of depression (Friedman, 1988). The preliminary findings that medications reduce autonomic arousal in PTSD patients lends support to the biological conceptualization of PTSD.

TREATMENT OF AUTONOMIC AROUSAL AND ANXIETY

Van der Kolk (1988) states:

> that autonomic arousal can be reduced at different levels in the central nervous system: through inhibition of the noradrenergic activity (clonidine and beta-adrenergic blockers), by increasing the inhibitory effect of the GABAergic system with GABAergic agonists (the benzodiazepines), and through the stabilization of the central nervous system...with lithium and carbamezapine. (p. 33)

Kolb, Burris, and Griffiths (1984) reported that using both clonidine and propranolol reduced intrusive experiences, startle response, explosiveness, and nightmare for chronic cases of PTSD. Van der Kolk (1988) reports that 14 of 22 patents on lithium report gaining a subjective sense of control over their lives. In particular, it was noted that the medication inhibited the "tendency to react to stress as if it were the recurrence of the original trauma" (p. 34).

In his review, Friedman, (1988) cited tricyclic antidepressants (especially imipramine) as reducing hyperarousal and intrusive reexperiences.

Hogben and Cornfield (1981) report success using phenelzine with patients demonstrating severe impairment, a chronic and deteriorating clinical course, and failure to respond to other treatment approaches, including other medications. Panic attacks were the most frequently occurring anxiety symptom among the subjects studied. In addition to reducing anxiety and physiological symptoms, phenelzine appeared to promote more successful involvement in therapy.

Friedman, (1988) suggests that phenelzine may be more appropriate with PTSD survivors who as a group (unlike Vietnam veterans) do not have drug and alcohol problems. These may be survivors of sexual trauma or natural disasters.

Benzodiazepines have been suggested as useful adjuncts for treating anxiety related to PTSD (van der Kolk, 1983; Yost, 1980.) Alpazolam (xanax) has been noted to be of particular interest because of its additional antipanic and antidepressant properties (Friedman, 1988). However, just about everyone cautions about the problems of these medications with PTSD patients who abuse drugs and alcohol (Friedman, 1988, van der Kolk 1988; Yost, 1980). In addition, Wise (1983) cautions that the benzodiazepines can often have a disinhibitory effect, potentially problematic with violent and aggressive patients.

SLEEP DISTURBANCES

Yost (1980) recommends the use of Dalmane for short-term sleep disorders. He emphasizes that barbituates should not be used, especially with Vietnam combat veterans with PTSD. "The risk of cross-tolerance with other drugs of addiction to which the veteran may have been exposed is too great to even consider these drugs useful in the condition" (p. 127). Kolb, Burris, and Griffiths (1984) note that clonidine and propranolol also promote improved sleep.

Roth (1988) suggests that use of triazolam (Halcion) over the use of Dalmane, because Dalmane's active metabolites have a 40-100 hour half-life. Van der Kolk (1988) anecdotally reports that amitriptyline has been reputed to be effective in treating chronic post-traumatic nightmares.

DEPRESSION

Tricyclic antidepressants are often used to treat the depressive symptomatology of PTSD patients (Friedman, 1988; Roth, 1988; Yost, 1980). Wise (1983) notes that antidepressant medication can be extremely helpful in cases where PTSD is compounded by serious depression. Hogben and Cornfield (1981) found improved patient motivation and more availability of affect with the use of the MAOI, phenelzine. However, Yost (1980) suggests that MAOIs should be used only rarely. When the individuals are suicidal, caution is advised.

PSYCHOTIC-LIKE SYMPTOMATOLOGY

Yost (1980) notes that only on rare occasions should antipsychotic medication be used with patients manifesting PTSD. He favors the use of antianxiety medications since the vast majority of psychotic-like phenomena are, with PTSD patients, really dissociative phenomena. When anti-psychotic medications are indicated, Yost (1980) recommends the use of high potency neuroleptic agents (at low doses) such as Haldol, Navane, and Loxitane. Friedman (1988) also argues that "anti-psychotic agents have no place in the routine treatment of PTSD" (p 283). Instead, he suggests reducing arousal with tricyclic antidepressants.

SUMMARY

At the present time the use of medication with PTSD is best considered an adjunctive treatment. Controlled studies on the use of psychoactive medications for treating PTSD are sorely needed. The essential indication for the use of medication is "when symptoms are so intense that they compromise working-through and adaptation rather than promoting them" (Roth, 1988, p. 41). Most authors strongly suggest that use of medication should not replace other therapeutic intervention; instead, it should enhance overall effectiveness of a broader therapeutic approach.

In addition, Roth (1988) has appropriately delineated several psychological issues associated with the psychopharmacological treatment of PTSD. At the outset of drug treatment, informed consent is particularly relevant for patients who have been traumatized. Without consent, the use of medication becomes one more situation in which something has been forced upon the patient. At the termination of drug treatment patients can feel relief, because it is proof that they are well again. For others, the termination of medication may be frightening, because it signals that society no longer considers them as "sick" as they feel. It can also lead to anger responses, displaced from authorities who failed to protect the victims to the doctors who failed to take their suffering seriously. With litigation pending, the withdrawal of medication can be viewed as a weakening of the case.

16

Summary

Upon reflection, we certainly hope the amount of information has not so overloaded the reader as to become a traumatic experience. This volume has been meant to serve as a clinical guide for mental health professionals interested in working with victims of trauma. If we have been successful the following goals should have been reached:

1. There should be little doubt in the reader's mind that PTSD exists as a psychological/psychiatric disorder.[23]
2. Readers should have a clear understanding of the primary and secondary symptoms of PTSD.
3. Readers should be aware of the view that human reaction to trauma tends to run a course with several possible end points.
4. Readers should understand the major theoretical formulations for understanding PTSD. They should also have an appreciation for the interaction of the different psychological variables that impact on the PTSD patient.
5. Clinicians will be better able to evaluate PTSD in both the clinical and forensic contexts.
6. Mental health providers will have a clearer understanding of the parameters involved in the therapy of PTSD. Clinicians will be more able to choose treatment modalities or integrate different modalities
7. Researchers should have a fuller appreciation of the important challenging questions to be addressed.

FUTURE TRENDS

It certainly probable that there will be a broadening of the contexts in which PTSD will be deemed relevant. Certainly, the experiences of rape and sexual abuse merit inclusion as stressors of severe enough proportions to meet DSM-IIIR criteria for trauma. Lengthy hospitalizations during early childhood may also be relevant contexts for assessing PTSD. There has already been a trend to associate unexpected loss, as through death of a loved one, with PTSD.

This latter context is an area that perhaps best fits another trend that is likely to develop in the next few years. Namely, it will be necessary to make sure that the construct of PTSD does not become too broad. There is likely to be an increasing sophistication in the diagnostic distinctions clinicians make. For instance, it really is not appropriate to say that the death of an 80-year-old father is an stressor beyond the realm of normal human experience.[24] However, the loss of a 5-year-old child may be considered beyond normal expectations, especially if the result of malfeasance or perceived carelessness.

Economic and political forces will remain strong influences in the field of PTSD. The increased sophistication of technology appears to lead to increasingly more elaborate disasters (e.g., TMI & Chernobyl). Under the Reagan administration there has been a lassitudinous attitude with regard to environmental protection as well as safety in the workplace. It is quite probable that these factors will result in more accidents, and therefore more diagnoses of PTSD. As PTSD becomes a more accepted diagnosis it is probable that it will be used more often in legal battles. As a result, two opposing trends may occur. One will be increased entrenchment on the part of insurance companies to limit payments by denying the existence or relevance of psychological factors in accidents (work-related or otherwise). The other possibility will be a realization that denying the problem does not make it go away. In this more progressive approach, primary and secondary prevention methods will be utilized to cut costs. It certainly may be necessary for clinical researchers to demonstrate the cost-effectiveness of early intervention for PTSD.

PREVENTION OF PTSD

Magelsdorf (1985) reported that as late as 1980 a planning report for natural disasters by the Pan American Health Organization stated that mental health problems secondary to disaster were not major acute public health problems. As research on the effect of trauma becomes more prevalent in quantity and quality, as well as becoming more a part of the general knowledge of clinicians, it is likely attention will shift to the prevention of PTSD in high risk-groups.

There is evidence that children are particularly susceptible to PTSD. There is also evidence that violence and the perception of imminent harm increase the probability of the development of PTSD. There is a belief (but as to date no clear research) that man-made disasters tend to cause more PTSD than natural disasters. There is also evidence that traumatized people with poor support systems are more likely to develop PTSD than traumatized individuals with good support systems.

Prevention Interventions

Once the high-risk groups have been defined, brief interventions can be designed to minimize the repercussions of the trauma. There are several types of intervention that would be useful.

Crisis Intervention. The basic tenets of crisis theory were discussed in Chapter 7. The most important axiom of crisis theory in understanding its usefulness in prevention is the concept that "a small external influence during a crisis state can produce disproportionate change in a short period of time when compared to therapeutic change that occurs during non-crisis states (Burgess & Baldwin, 1981, p.31). In other words, along an individual's path of development, a crisis serves as a nexus. The trajectory taken from the nexus can cause profound differences in the path of development taken. One has the most therapeutic leverage at the point of crisis.

Stress Inoculation Training. Stress Inoculation Training would seem to be uniquely useful as prevention approach when severe stress is likely to be known ahead of time. The successful use of this strategy with Israeli children who were repeatedly being shelled was reported in Chapter 10. It would be interesting to compare soldiers going into battle who had a course of S.I.T. versus those who did not. S.I.T would also be useful as an early intervention approach after trauma.

CHANGES IN THEORY

The disagreement over whether or not to place PTSD under dissociative disorders or anxiety disorders in the DSM-IIIR has already been mentioned. We suspect that the dissociative aspects of PTSD may gain in prominence as an explanatory principle of the disorder. We have purposefully kept the Pandora's box of the similarity between PTSD and multiple personality disorder closed. Eventually the implications of the commonalities of these disorders needs to be discussed more fully in the literature.

Another change that is likely to be important is the study of how people stay healthy in spite of trauma. Of course, this shift from a pathology paradigm to a health paradigm is gradually occurring throughout the mental health field. The specificity of the stressor with resultant adaptation or maladaptation makes this category of disorder a prime candidate for looking at these issues.

CHANGES IN ASSESSMENT

The change that most needs to occur is the standardization of the evaluation of PTSD. It is likely that this development will occur. Horowitz (personal communication, June 1988) is in the process of expanding the norms of the Impact of Events Scale. The PTSD scale of the MMPI needs further validation and cross-validation. Unfortunately, the MMPI has mostly been used on combat-related PTSD. It would be useful to have information on other types of PTSD populations. Furthermore, such data may help settle the issue of whether or not an elevated F-scale is indicative of the severe emotional distress common with the disorder or if it is an indication of exaggeration of symptoms. A related issue, is whether or not there are significant differences in the assessment or the treatment of PTSD stemming from different types of stressors.

CHANGES IN THERAPY

In recent years there has been an increasing interest in the use of brief therapy (Budman & Gurman, 1988; de Shazer, 1985, 1988). This trend has already existed for the treatment of stress reactions, and is likely to continue. There will probably be an increasing pressure to demonstrate treatment efficacy. This is part of a general trend in the mental health field. There certainly is a need for better methodology in psychotherapy outcome research (in the PTSD arena, and in other areas as well). Although there is no evidence to support this claim, we would like to suggest that PTSD is an excellent diagnostic entity to use for psychotherapy research. The reason that it may be of particular use is that there is a discrete stressor. Given the likelihood that the incidence of individuals suffering from PTSD will increase, there is a need for clinicians and researchers to turn their attention to this important problem. This book is one small effort to help alleviate the stress of those who have been traumatized.

Notes

CHAPTER 2

1. As required by the DSM-III-R for the diagnosis of PTSD.
2. Survivor guilt was described in the DSM-III as "guilt about surviving when others have not, or about behavior required for survival" (APA, 1980, p. 238).

CHAPTER 4

3. Once again, we want to emphasize the heuristic nature of stage conceptualization.

CHAPTER 5

4. The reaction index was standardized on 750 children and 1350 adults. The validity correlations with known cases of PTSD was 0.91 among children and 0.95 among adults (Frederick, 1985).
5. Denial and massive repression are operationally defined to mean that the person cannot remember, even when trying. This is different from suppression, in which the incident may be out of consciousness, but can be accurately recalled with effort.
6. Familicide is the attempted murder of all the members of a family.

CHAPTER 6

7. A more complete treatment goal would be to initiate an adaptive deviation-amplification circuit.
8. Several variables will not be discussed in any detail, because we have nothing new to contribute. These include Post-traumatic cognitive processing, the recovery environment, and individual characteristics.

CHAPTER 7

9. A color-form response is based primarily on color aspects of the blot, and also includes some reference to form (Exner, 1974).
10. The human movement response is scored when the person sees human activity in the blot (Exner, 1974).
11. *Early morning awakening with difficulty returning to sleep.*
12. The F-scale is generally thought of as a measure of subjects' tendency to exaggerate the difficulties they are experiencing. High scores, above 90, represent malingering or a plea for help or random responding (Greene, 1980).
13. These categories are often cited by other authors as well.
14. We would like to acknowledge Jan Grossman, Ph. D., and Rae Maybon, J.D., for their help in delineating the issues in this section.
15. The alpha level is the probability criterion that is set ahead of time for rejecting the null hypothesis. In the social sciences an alpha level of 0.05 is the minimum criterion. This means that if the chance of the outcome is 1 in 20 or less, it is probably not due to chance.
16. We would like to thank Jan Grossman, Ph. D., for describing this line of questioning.
17. The implication of this sentence is to try yet fail.

CHAPTER 11

18. This formulation complements the formulations by Epstein (1990) and Janoff-Bulman (1983)
19. Although some of the group members probably met DSM-III-R criteria for PTSD.
20. A less hypnotizable person can also benefit from hypnosis. However, the therapist usually needs to be more indirect and more creative. Even persons at extremely low levels of hypnotizability can benefit from indirect and permissive hypnotic approaches. In any event, PTSD patients tend to be highly hypnotizable.

21. While it is not important that the therapist know the content of what will happen, if the therapist does not have any sense of the type of *process* that the patient will exhibit, hypnosis should be reserved until such time as the therapist has a sense of how the patient will respond to the trance.

CHAPTER 14

22. With the Rutter Behavioral Questionnaire.

References

Adams, M.F. (1982). PTSD: An inpatient treatment unit. *American Journal of Nursing,* 82 (11), 1704–1705.

Alberti, R.E., & Emmons, M.L. (1978). *Your perfect right: A guide to assertive behavior (3rd ed.).* San Luis Obispo, CA: Impact.

Alexander, J.F., & Parsons, B.V. (1981). *Functional family therapy: Principles and procedures.* Monterey, CA: Brooks/Cole.

American Psychiatric Association (1952). *Diagnostic and statistical manual.* Washington D.C.: Author.

American Psychiatric Association (1968). *Diagnostic and statistical manual* (2nd ed). Washington D.C.: Author.

American Psychiatric Association (1980). *Diagnostic and statistical manual of mental disorders* (3rd ed.) Washington DC: Author.

American Psychiatric Association (1987). Diagnostic and statistical manual of mental disorders (3rd ed.-revised) Washington DC: Author.

Archibald, H.C., Long, D.M., Miller, C., & Tuddenham, R.D. (1962). Gross stress reaction in combat—A 15-year follow-up. *American Journal of Psychiatry,* 119, 317–322.

Archibald, H.C., & Tuddenham, R.D. (1965). Persistent stress reactions after combat: A 20-year follow-up. *Archives of General Psychiatry,* 12, 475–481.

Arnold, A.L. (1985a). Diagnosis of post-traumatic stress disorder in Vietnam veterans. In S.M. Sonnenberg, A.S. Blank, J.A. Talbott (Eds.), *The trauma of war: Stress and recovery in Vietnam veterans* (99–124). Washington, DC: American Psychiatric Press.

Arnold, A.L. (1985b). Inpatient treatment of Vietnam veterans with post-traumatic stress disorder. In S.M. Sonnenberg, A.S. Blank, J.A. Talbott (Eds.), *The trauma of war: Stress and recovery in Vietnam veterans* (pp. 239–262). Washington, DC: American Psychiatric Press.

Araoz, D. L. (1985) *The new hypnosis.* New York: Brunner/Mazel.

Arryo, B. & Eth, S. (1985). Children traumatized by Central American warfare. In S. Eth & R. Pynoos (Eds.) *Post-traumatic stress disorder in children.* Washington, DC: American Psychiatric Press.

Atkinson, R.M., Henderson, R.G., Sparr, L.R., & Peale, S. (1982). Assessment of Vietnam veterans for post-traumatic stress disorder in veterans administrations disability claims. *American Journal of Psychiatry,* 139 (9), 1118–1121.

Ayalon, O. (1983). Coping with terrorism. In D. Meichenbaum & M. Jaremko (Eds.), *Stress reduction and prevention.* New York: Plenum.

Bailey, J.E. (1985). Differential diagnosis of posttraumatic stress and antisocial personality disorders. *Hospital and Community Psychiatry,* 36 (8), 881–883.

Baker, E. L. (1985). Hypnosis with psychotic and borderline patients. In B. Zilbergeld, M. G. Edelstein, D. L. Araoz (Eds.), *Hypnosis questions and answers.* New York: Norton.

Balson, P.M. (1980). Treatment of war neuroses from Vietnam. *Comprehensive Psychiatry,* 21 (2), 167–175.

Bandura, A. (1971). Psychotherapy based on modeling principles. In S.E. Bergin & S.L. Garfield (Eds.). *Handbook of psychotherapy and behavior change.* New York: Wiley.

Bandura, A. (1977). Self-efficacy: Toward a unifying theory of behavioral change. *Psychological Review, 84,* 191–215.

Bandura, A. (1982). Self-efficacy mechanism in human agency. *American Psychologist, 37,* 122–147.

Baum, A., Gratchel. R.J., & Schaeffer, M.A. (1983). Emotional,behavioral, and physiological effects of chronic stress at Three Mile Island. *Journal of Clinical and Consulting Psychology,* 51 (4), 488–494.

Beck, A. T. (1967). *Depression: Clinical, experimental, and theoretical aspects.* New York: Harper & Row.

Ben-Eli, T., & Sela, M. (1980). Terrorists in Nahariya: Description of coping under stress (Hebr.). *Israeli Journal of Psychology and Counselling in Education,* 13, 94–101.

Belliveay, F., & Richter, L. (1970). *Understanding human sexual inadequacy.* New York: Bantam Books.

Benson, H. (1975). *The relaxation response.* New York: Avon Books.

Berger, D.M. (1977). The survivor syndrome: A problem of nosology and treatment. *American Journal of Psychotherapy,* 31 (2), 238–251.

Berkowitz, M. (1980). Themes in treatment of Vietnam veterans. In: T. Williams (Ed.). *Post-traumatic stress disorders of Vietnam veterans* (133–135). Cincinnatti, OH: Disabled American Veterans.

Bernstein, A.D., & Borkoec, T.D. (1973). *Progressive relaxation training: A manual for the helping professions.* Champaign, IL: Research Press.

Bertalanffy, L. von (1968). *General systems theory: Foundations, development, applications.* New York: George Braziller.

Berzoff, J. (1974). A review of the literature on survival of persecution and the after-effects of massive traumatization. *Smith College Studies in Social Work,* 45 (1), 42–43.

Bey, D.R., & Zecchenelli, V.A. (1971). Marijuana as a coping device in Vietnam. *Military Medicine,* 136, 448–450.

Birkhimer, L.J., DeVane, C.L., & Muniz, C.E. (1985). Post-traumatic stress disorder: Characteristics and pharmacological response in the veteran population. *Comprehensive Psychiatry,* 26 (3), 304–310.

Blanchard, E.B., Kolb, L.C., Pallmeyer, B.A., & Gerardi, R.J. (1982). A psychophysiological study of post-traumatic stress disorder in Vietnam veterans. *Psychiatric Quarterly,* 54 (4), 220–229.

Blank, A.S. (1985a). Irrational reactions to post-traumatic stress disorder and Vietnam veterans. In S.M. Sonnenberg, A.S. Blank, J.A. Talbott (Eds.), *The trauma of war: Stress and recovery in Vietnam veterans* (pp. 69–98). Washington, DC: American Psychiatric Press.

Blank, A.S. (1985b). The unconscious flashback to the war in Vietnam veterans: Clinical mystery, legal defense, and community problem. In S.M. Sonnenberg, A.S. Blank,

J.A. Talbott (Eds.), *The trauma of war: Stress and recovery in Vietnam veterans* (pp. 293–308). Washington, DC: American Psychiatric Press.

Bloch, G.R., & Bloch, N.H. (1976). Analytic group psychotherapy of post-traumatic psychoses. *International Journal of Group Psychotherapy, 26,* (1), 49–57.

Block, J.H., & Block, J. (1978). *The role of ego-control and ego-resiliency in the organization of behavior.* New York: Lawrence Erlbaum.

Boehnlein, J.K., Kinzie, J.D., Ben, R., & Fleck, J. (1985). One-year follow-up study of post-traumatic stress disorder among survivors of Cambodian concentration camps. *American Journal of Psychiatry, 142* (8), 956–959.

Bourne, P.G. (1970 a). Military psychiatry and the Vietnam experience. *American Journal of Psychiatry, 127,* 481–488.

Bourne, P.G. (1970 b). *Men, stress, and Vietnam.* Boston: Little, Brown.

Bourne, P.G. (1972). The Vietnam veteran. *Psychiatry in Medicine, 3,* 23–27.

Borus, J.F. (1973). Re-entry: III. Facilitating healthy readjustment in Vietnam veterans. *Psychiatry, 36,* 428–439.

Borus, J.F. (1974). Incidence of maladjustment in Vietnam returnees. *Archives of General Psychiatry, 30,* 554–557.

Bowen, M. (1976). Theory in the practice of psychotherapy. In M. Bowen (Ed.). *Family Therapy in clinical practice* (337–388). New York: Jason Aronson.

Bowen, M. (Ed.) (1978). *Family therapy in clinical practice.* New York: Jason Aronson.

Braceland, F.J. (1982). Personal reflections: Forgotten men. *Psychiatric Annals, 12,* 975–976.

Brende, J.O. (1981). Combined individual and group therapy for Vietnam veterans. *International Journal of Group Psychotherapy, 31* (3), 367–377.

Brende, J.O. (1982). Electrodermal responses in post-traumatic stress disorders. *Journal of Nervous and Mental Diseases, 170* (6), 352–356.

Brende, J.O. (1983). A psychodynamic view of character pathology in Vietnam combat veterans. *Bulletin of the Menninger Clinic, 47* (3), 193–210.

Brende, J.O. (1985). The use of hypnosis in post-traumatic conditions. In W.E. Kelly (Ed.), *Post-traumatic stress disorder and the war veteran patient* (pp. 193–210). New York: Brunner/Mazel.

Brende, J.O., & Benedict, B.D. (1980). The Vietnam combat delayed stress syndrome: Hypnotherapy of "dissociative symptoms." *American Journal of Clinical Hypnosis, 23,* 34–40.

Brende, J.O., & McCann, I.L. (1984). Regressive experience in Vietnam veterans: Their relationship to war, post-traumatic symptoms, and recovery. *Journal of Contemporary Psychiatry, 14,* 57–75.

Breslau, N. & Davis, G. C. (1987). Posttraumatic stress disorder: The etiological specificity of wartime stressors. *American Journal of Psychiatry, 144* (5), 578–582.

Brett, E.A. (1985). Imagery and posttraumatic stress disorder: An overview. *American Journal of Psychiatry, 142* (4), 417–424.

Breuer, J., & Freud, S. (1895/1955). *Studies in hysteria. Standard Edition, Vol. II.* London: Hogarth Press.

Budman, S. H., & Gurman, A. S. (1988). *Theory and practice of brief therapy.* New York: Guilford Press.

Bullman, R. J., & Wortman C. B. (1977). Atributions of blame and coping in the "real world": Severe accident victims react to their lot. *Journal of Personality and Social Psychology, 35,* 351–363.

Burgess, A.W., & Baldwin, B.A. (1981). *Crisis intervention theory and practice: A clinical handbook.* Englewood Cliffs, NJ: Prentice-Hall.

Burgess, A.W., & Holmstrom, L.L. (1974). Rape trauma syndrome. *American Journal of Psychiatry, 131* (9), 981–986.

Burgess, A.W., & Holmstrom, L.L. (1976). Coping behavior of the rape victim. *American Journal of Psychiatry*, 133 (4), 413–417.

Burgess, A.W., & Holmstrom, L.L. (1979). *Rape: Crisis and recovery.* Bowie, MD: Robert J. Brady.

Bychowski, G. (1968). *Evil in man: Anatomy of hate and violence.* New York: Grune & Stratton.

Caplan, G. (1961). *Principles of preventive psychiatry.* New York: Basic Books.

Caren, E. (H.), Rieker, P.P., & Mills, T. (1984). Victims of violence and psychiatric illness. *American Journal of Psychiatry*, 141 (3), 378–383.

Carter, J.H. (1982). Alcoholism in black Vietnam veterans: Symptoms of PTSD. *Journal of the National Medical Association*, 74 (7), 655–660.

Cone, J.D., & Hawkins, R.P. (1977). *Behavioral assessment: New directions in clinical psychology.* New York: Brunner/Mazel.

Cowtela, J.R., & Kastenbaum, R.A. (1967). A reinforcement schedule for use in therapy, training, and research. *Psychological Reports*, 20, 1115–1130.

Cavenar, J.O. (1976). The effects of combat on the normal personality: War neurosis in Vietnam veterans. *Comprehensive Psychiatry*, 17 (5), 647–653.

Celluci, A.J., & Lawrence. P.S. (1978). The efficacy of systematic desensitization in reducing nightmares. *Journal of Behavior Therapy and Experimental Psychiatry*, 9, 109–114.

Christenson, R.M., Walker, J.I., Ross, D.R., & Moltbie, A.A. (1981). Reactivation of traumatic conflicts. *American Journal of Psychiatry*, 138 (7), 984–985.

Corcoran, J.F.T. (1982). The concentration camp syndrome and USAF Vietnam prisoners of war. *Psychiatric Annals*, 12 (11), 991–994.

Danieli, Y. (1985). The treatment and prevention of long-term effects and intergenerational transmission of victimization: A lesson from holocaust survivors and their children. In C.R. Figley (Ed.), *Trauma and its wake: The study and the treatment of posttraumatic stress disorder* (295–313). New York: Brunner/Mazel.

Davidson, L.M., & Baum, A. (1986). Chronic stress and posttraumatic disorders. *Journal of Consulting and Clinical Psychology*, 54, (3) 303–308.

DeFazio, V.J. (1975). The Vietnam era veteran: Psychological problems. *Journal of Contemporary Psychotherapy*, 7 (1), 9–15.

DeFazio, V.J. (1978). Dynamic perspectives on the nature and effects of combat stress. In C.R. Figley (Ed.), *Stress disorders among Vietnam veterans: Theory, research, and practice.* New York: Brunner/Mazel.

de la Penna, A. (1984) PTSD in the Vietnam vet: A brain-modulated, compensator, information-augmenting response to information underload in the CNS. In B. A. van der Kolk (Ed.), *PTSD: Psychological and biological sequelae.* Washington DC: American Psychiatric Press.

de Shazer, S. (1985). *Keys to solution in brief therapy.* New York: Norton.

de Shazer, S. (1988). *Clues to solution in brief therapy.* New York: Norton.

Dobbs, D., & Wilson, W. P. (1960). Observations on the persistence of war neurosis. *Diseases of the nervous system*, 21, 686–691.

Dollard, J., & Miler, N. E. (1950). *Personality and Psychotherapy.* New York: McGraw-Hill

Domash, M.D., & Sparr, L.F. (1982). Post-traumatic stress disorder masquerading as paranoid schizophrenia: Case report. *Military Medicine*, 147, 772–774.

D'Zurilla, T.J., & Goldfried, M.R. (1971). Problem solving and behavior modification. *Journal of Abnormal Psychology*, 78, 107–126.

Early, P. (1982). Nurses haunted by memories of service in Vietnam. *American Nurse*, 14 (2), 8.

Egendorf, A. (1978). Psychotherapy with Vietnam veterans: Observations and suggestions. In C.R. Figley (Ed.). *Stress disorders among Vietnam veterans: theory, research, and practice.* New York: Brunner/Mazel.

Eitinger, L. (1971). Organic and psychosomatic aftereffects of concentration camp imprisonment. In H. Krystal and W. G. Niederland, (Eds.). *Psychic traumatization.* Boston: Little, Brown.

Ellis, A. (1962). *Reason and emotion in psychotherapy.* New York: Lyle Stuart.

Enzie, R.F., Sawyer, R.N., & Montgomery, F.A. (1973). Manifest anxiety of Vietnam returnees and undergraduates. *Psychological Reports, 33*, 446.

Epstein, A.W. (1982). Mental phenomena across generations: The holocaust. *Journal of the American Academy of Psychoanalysis, 10* (4), 565–570.

Epstein, S. (1990). Beliefs and symptoms in maladaptive resolutions of the traumatic neurosis. In D. Ozer, J.M. Healy & A.J. Stewart (Eds.), *Perspectives on personality, Vol. 3.* London: Jessica Kingsley, Publishers.

Erikson, E. (1946). Ego development and historical change: Clinical notes. *Psychoanalytic Study of the Child, 2*, 379–389.

Erikson, E. (1968). *Youth, identity, and crisis.* New York: Norton.

Erikson, K.T. (1976). Loss of communality at Buffalo Creek. *American Journal of Psychiatry, 133* (3), 302–305.

Erikson, M.H. (1959). Further clinical techniques of hypnosis: Utilization techniques. *The American Journal of Clinical Hypnosis, 2*, 3–21.

Erickson, M.H., & Kubie, L.S. (1941). Successful treatment of a case of acute hysterical depression by return under hypnosis to critical phase of childhood. *Psychoanalytic Quarterly, 10*, 583–699.

Erickson, M. H., & Rossi, E. L. (1979). *Hypnotherapy: An exploratory casebook.* New York: Irvington.

Eysenk, H.J. (1976). The learning theory model of neurosis—A new approach. *Behavior Research and Therapy, 14*, 251–267.

Fairbank, J.A., DeGood, D.E., & Jenkins, C.W. (1981). Behavioral treatment of a persistent post-traumatic response. *Journal of Behavioral Therapy and Experiemental Psychiatry, 12* (4), 321–324.

Fairbank, J.A., & Keane, T. M. (1982). Flooding for combat-related stress disorders: Assessment of anxiety reduction across traumatic memories. *Behavior Therapy, 13*, 499–510.

Fairbank, J.A., Keane, T.M., & Malloy, P.F. (1983). Some preliminary data on the psychological characteristics of Vietnam veterans with posttraumatic stress disorders. *Journal of Clinical and Consulting Psychology, 51* (6), 912–919.

Fairbank, J.A., Langley, K., Jarvine, G.J., & Keane, T.M. (1981). A selected bibliography on posttraumatic stress disorders in Vietnam veterans. *Professional psychology, 12* (5), 578–586.

Fairbank. J. A.. McCaffrey, R., & Keane, T. M. (1985). Psychometric detection of fabricated symptoms of PTSD. *American Journal of Psychiatry, 142*, 501–503.

Fenichel, O. (1946). *The psychoanalytic theory of neurosis.* New York: Norton.

Fensterheim, H., & Baer, J. (1975). *Don't say yes when you want to say no.* New York: Dell.

Figley, C.R. (1977). *The American Legion study of psychological adjustment among Vietnam veterans. Lafayette, IN: Purdue University.*

Figley, C.R. (Ed.) (1978). *Stress disorders among Vietnam veterans: Theory, research, and practice.* New York: Brunner/Mazel.

Figley, C.R. (Ed.) (1985). *Trauma and its wake: The study and treatment of post-traumatic stress disorder.* New York: Brunner/Mazel.

Figley, C. R. (1988). Post-traumatic family therapy. In F. Ochberg (Ed.) *Post-traumatic therapy and victims of violence.* New York: Brunner/Mazel.

Figley, C.R., & Leventman, S. (Eds.) (1980). *Strangers at home: Vietnam veterans since the war.* New York: Praeger.

Figley, C.R., & Spenkle, D.H. (1978). Delayed stress response syndrome: Family therapy indications. *Journal of Marriage and Family Counselling,* 4, 53–59.

Fogelman, E., & Sauran, B. (1980). Brief group therapy with offspring of holocaust survivors: Leader's reactions. *American Journal of Orthopsychiatry,* 50 (1), 96–108.

Forman, B.D. (1980). Psychotherapy with rape victims. *Psychotherapy: Theory, research, and practice,* 17 (3), 304–311.

Foy, D.W., Sipprelle, R.C., Rueger, D.B., & Carroll, E.M. (1984). Etiology of posttraumatic stress disorder in Vietnam veterans: Analysis of premilitary, military, and combat exposure influences. *Journal of Clinical and Consulting Psychology,* 52 (1), 79–87.

Frank, E., Turner, S.M., Stewart, B.D., Jacob, M., & West, D. (1981). Past psychiatric symptoms and the response to sexual assault. *Comprehensive Psychiatry,* 22 (5), 479–487.

Frederick, C. J. (1985b). Selected foci in the spectrum of post-traumatic stress disorders. In S. Murphy & J. Laube (Eds.) *Perspectives on disaster recovery.* New York: Appleton-Century-Crofts.

Frederick, C. J. (1987). Psychic trauma in victims of crime and terrorism. in G.R. VandenBos & B.K. Bryant (Eds.) *Cataclysm, crises and catastrophes: Psychology in action-master Lecture Series.* Washington, DC: American Psychological Association.

Free fire zone: Stories by Vietnam veterans (1975). Brooklyn: First Casualty Press.

Freud, A., & Burlingame, D. (1943). *Children and war.* New York: Ernst Willard.

Freud, S. (1919). *Introduction to the psychology of the war neuroses.* Standard Edition, 18. London: Hogarth Press.

Freud, S. (1920/1955). *Beyond the pleasure principle.* Standard Edition 18. London: Hogarth Press.

Freud, S., Ferenczi, K., Abraham, K., & Jones, E. (1921). *Psychoanalysis and the war neuroses.* New York: International Psychoanalytic Press.

Frick, R., & Bogart, L. (1982). Transference and countertransference in group therapy with Vietnam veterans. *Bulletin of the Menninger Clinic,* 46 (5), 429–444.

Friedman, M. J. (1988). Toward rational pharmacotherapy for posttraumatic stress disorder: An interim report. *American Journal of Psychiatry,* 145 (3), 281–285 .

Frye, J.S., & Stockton, R.A. (1982). Discriminant analysis of posttraumatic stress disorder among a group of Vietnam veterans. *American Journal of Psychiatry,* 139 (1), 52–56.

Fuentes, R. (1980). Therapist transparency. In T. Williams (Ed.). *Posttraumatic stress disorders of the Vietnam veteran* (pp. 137–138). Cincinnatti, OH: Disabled American Veterans.

Furst, S. (Ed.) (1967). *Psychic trauma.* New York: Basic Books.

Futterman, S., & Pumpion-Mindlin, E. (1951). Traumatic war neuroses for five years later. *American Journal of Psychiatry,* 108, 401–408.

Galante, R., & Foa, D. (1986). An epidemiological study of psychic trauma and treatment effectiveness for children after a natural disaster. *Journal of the American Academy of Child Psychiatry,* 25, 357–363.

Geer, J.H., & Silverman, J. (1967). Treatment of a recurrent nightmare by behavior modification procedures. *Journal of Abnormal Psychology,* 72, 188–190.

Gelfand, D.M., & Hartmann, D.P. (1975). *Child behavior analysis and therapy.* New York: Pergamon.

Galassi, J.P., Delo, J.S., Galassi, M.D., & Bastren, S. (1974). The college self-expression scale: A measure of assertiveness. *Behavior Therapy,* 5, 165–171.

Gilligan. S. G., and Kennedy, C. E. (in press). Solutions and resolutions: Ericksonian hypnotherapy with incest survivor groups. *Journal of Strategic and Systemic Therapy*

Goldfrield, M.R.. (1972). Systematic desensitization as training in self control. *Journal of Consulting and Clinical Psychology,* 37, 228–234.

Goldfrield, M.R., & Davidson, G.C. (1976). *Clinical behavior therapy.* New York: Holt, Rinehart, and Winston.

Goldfrield, M.R., & Trier, C.S. (1974). Effectiveness of relaxation as an active coping skill. *Journal of Abnormal Psychology,* 83, 348–355.

Goodwin, J. (1980). The etiology of combat-related post-traumatic stress disorders. In T. Williams (Ed.). *Posttraumatic stress disorders of the Vietnam veteran* (1–23). Cincinnati, OH: Disabled American Veterans.

Goodwin, D.W., Davis, D.H., & Robins, L.N. (1975). Drinking among abundant illicit drugs. *Archives of General Psychiatry,* 32, 230–233.

Graham, J. (1977). *The MMPI: Practical guide.* New York: Oxford University Press.

Green, B.L., Grace, M.C., Lindy, J.D., Titchener, J.L., & Lindy, J.G. (1983). Levels of functional impairment following a civilian disaster: The Beverly Hills Supper Club fire. *Journal of Clinical and Consulting Psychology,* 51 (4), 573–580.

Green B. L., Wilson, J. P., and Lindy J. D. (1985). Conceptualizing post-traumatic stress disorder: A psychosocial framework. in C. R. Figley (Ed.) *Trauma and its wake: The study and treatment of post-traumatic stress disorder.* New York: Brunner/Mazel.

Greenberg, M. S., & van der Kolk, B. A. (1986). Retrieval and integration of traumatic memories with the "painting cure." in B. A. van der Kolk (eds.) *Psychological Trauma.* Washington, DC: American Psychiatric Press.

Greenstone, J.L., & Leviton, S.C. (1981). Crisis management. In R.J. Corsini (Ed.), *Handbook of Innovative Psychotherapies* (216–228). New York: John Wiley & Sons.

Grinker, R.R., & Spiegel, J.P. (1945). *War neuroses.* Philadelphia: Blakiston.

Groesbeck, C.J. (1982). Dreams of a Vietnam veteran—A Jungian perspective. *Psychiatric Annals,* 12 (11), 1007–1008.

Haley, J. (1973). *Uncommon therapy: The psychiatric technique of Milton H. Erikson, M.D.* New York: Norton.

Haley, J. (1976). *Problem-solving therapy.* San Francisco: Jossey-Bass.

Haley, S.A. (1974). When the patient reports atrocities: Specific treatment considerations of the Vietnam veteran. *Archives of General Psychiatry,* 30, 191–196.

Haley, S.A. (1978). Treatment implications of post-combat stress response syndromes for mental health professionals. In C.R. Figley (Ed.), *Stress disorders among Vietnam veterans: Theory, research, and practice* (254–267). New York: Brunner/Mazel.

Haley, S.A. (1985). Some of my best friends are dead: Treatment of the PTSD patient and his family. In W.E. Kelly (Ed.), *Post-traumatic stress disorder and the war veteran patient* (54–71). New York: Brunner/Mazel.

Hamilton, J. W. (1982). Unusual long-term sequelae of a traumatic war experience. *Bulletin of the Menninger Clinic,* 46 (6), 539–541.

Hanford, H. A., Dickerson Mayers, S., Mattison, R. E., Humphrey, F. J., Bagnato, S., Bixler, E. O. & Kales, J. D. (1986). Child and parent reactions to the three mile island nuclear accident. *Journal of the American Academy of Child Psychiatry,* 25, (3), 346–356.

Hassener, P.W., and McCary, P.W. (1974). A comparative study of the attitudes of veterans and nonveterans at the University of Northern Colorado. *Colorado Journal of Educational Research,* 14, 11–18.

Hellekson, E.C. (1981). Posttraumatic stress disorder of a former hostage (letter). *American Journal of Psychiatry,* 138 (7), 991.

Hendin, H. (1983). Psychotherapy for Vietnam veterans with post-traumatic stress disorders. *American Journal of Psychotherapy,* 37 (1), 86–99.

Hendin, H. (1984). Combat never ends: The paranoid adaptation to posttraumatic stress. *American Journal of Psychotherapy,* 38 (1), 121–131.

Hendin, H., and Haas, A. P. (1984). *Wounds of War: The psychological aftermath of combat in Vietnam.* New York: Basic Books.

Hendin, H., Pollinger Hass, A., Singer, Houghton, W., Schwartz, M., & Wallen, V. (1984). The reliving experience in Vietnam veterans with posttraumatic stress disorder. *Comprehensive Psychiatry*, 25 (2), 165–173.

Hendin, H., Pollinger, A., Singer, P., & Ulman, R.B. (1981). Meanings of combat and the development of posttraumatic stress disorder. *American Journal of Psychiatry*, 138 (11), 1490–1493.

Hilgard, E. R. (1974). Toward a neodissociation theory: Multiple cognitive controls in human functioning. *Perspectives in Biology and Medicine*, 17, 301–316.

Hillman, R.G. (1981). The psychopathology of being held a hostage. *American Journal of Psychiatry*, 138 (9), 1193–1197.

Hoffman, L.E. (1981). War, revolution, and psychoanalysis: Freudian thought begins to grapple with social reality. *Journal of the History of the Behavioral Sciences*, 17 (2), 251–269.

Hogben, G.L., and Cornfield, R.B. (1981). Treatment of traumatic war neurosis with phenelzine. *Archives of General Psychiatry*, 38, 440–445.

Holmstrom, L.L., and Burgess, A.W. (1975). Assessing trauma in the rape victim. *American Journal of Nursing*, 75 (8), 1288–1291.

Hoppe, K.D. (1971). The aftermath of Nazi persecution reflected in recent psychiatric literature. In H. Krystal and W.G. Niederland (Eds.). *Psychic traumatization*. Boston: Little, Brown.

Horowitz, M.J. (1973). Phase-oriented treatment of stress response syndromes. *American Journal of Psychotherapy*, 27, 506–515.

Horowitz, M.J. (1974). Stress response syndromes: Character style and dynamic psychotherapy. *Archives of General Psychiatry*, 31, 768–781.

Horowitz, M.J. (1976). *Stress response syndromes*. New York: Jason Aronson.

Horowitz, M.J. (1979). Psychological response to serious life events. In V. Hamilton and D.M. Warburton (Eds.). *Human stress and cognition*. New York: Wiley.

Horowitz, M.J. (1983). *Image formation and psychotherapy* (rev. ed.). New York: Jason Aronson.

Horowitz, M.J. (1986). *Stress response syndromes* (2nd ed.). New York: Jason Aronson.

Horowitz, M.J., & Solomon G.F. (1975). A prediction of delayed stress response syndromes in Vietnam veterans. *Journal of Social Issues*, 4, 67–80.

Horowitz, M.J., & Solomon, G.F. (1978). Delayed stress response syndromes in Vietnam veterans. In C.R. Figley (Ed.), *Stress response syndromes among Vietnam veterans: Theory, research, and practice* (pp. 268–280). New York: Brunner/Mazel.

Horowitz, M.J., & Wilner, N. (1976). Stress films, emotion, and cognitive repsonse. *Archives of General Psychiatry*, 33, 1339–1344.

Horowitz, M.J., Wilner, N., Kaltreider, N., & Alvarez, M.A. (1980). Signs and symptoms of posttraumatic stress disorder. *Archives of General Psychiatry*, 37, 85–92.

Horowitz, M.J., Wilner, N., Marmar, C., & Krupnick, J. (1980). Pathological grief and the activation of latent self-images. *American Journal of Psychiatry*, 137 (10), 1157–1162.

Howard, S. (1976). The Vietnam warrior: His experience and implications for psychotherapy. *American Journal of Psychotherapy*, — —, 121–135.

Hugett, W.T. (1973). The body count. New York: Putnam.

Hyer, L., Fallon, J. H., Harrison, W., & Boudewyns (1987). MMPI overreporting by Vietnam veterans. *Journal of Clinical Psychology*, 43, 79–83.

Hyer, L., O'leary. W., Saucer, R., Blount, J., Harrison, W., & Boudewyns (1986). Inpatient diagnosis of posttraumatic stress disorder. *Journal of Consulting and Clinical Psychology*, 54, 698–702

Jacobson, E. (1938). *Progressive relaxation*. Chicago: University of Chicago Press.

Jaffe, R. (1968). Dissociative phenomena in former concentration camp inmates. *International Journal of Psychoanalysis*, 49 (3), 310–312.

Janis, I. L (1983) Stress inoculation in health care: Theory and research. In D. Meichenbaum & M. Jaremko (Eds). *Stress reduction and prevention*. New York: Plenum.

Janoff-Bulman, R. (1985). The aftermath of victimization: Rebuilding shattered assumptions. In C. R. Figley (Ed.), *Trauma and its wake: The study and treatment of post-traumatic stress disorder*. New York: Brunner/Mazel.

Jung, C.G. (1954). Therpeutic value of abreaction. In *The practice of psychotherapy, Collected Works, Vol. XVI*. Princeton, NJ: Princeton University Press.

Jurich, A.P. (1983). The Saigon of the family's mind: Family therapy with families of Vietnam veterans. *Journal of Marital and Family Therapy*, 9 (4), 355–363.

Kahana, R.J. (1981). The aging survivor of the holocaust. *Journal of Geriatric Psychiatry*, 14 (2), 225–239.

Kalinowski, L.B. (1950). Problems of war neroses in the light of experiences in other countries. *American Journal of Psychiatry*, 107, 340–346.

Kardiner, A. (1941). *The traumatic neuroses of war*. New York: Hoeber.

Kardiner. A. (1959). Traumatic neurosis of war. In S. Arieti (Ed.). *American handbook of psychiatry*. New York: Basic Books.

Keane, T. M., Malloy, P. F., & Fairbank, J.A. (1984). Empirical development of an MMPI subscale for the assessment of combat-related PTSD. *Journal of Consulting and Clinical Psychology*, 62, 888–891.

Keane, T. M., Fairbank, J.A., Caddell, R. T., Zimering, R. T., & Bender, M. E. (1985). A behavioral approach to assessing and treating PTSD in Vietnam veterans. In C. R. Figley (Ed.) *Trauma and its wake*. New York: Brunner/Mazel.

Keane, T.M., & Fairbank, J.A. (1983). Survey analysis of combat related stress disorders in Vietnam veterans. *American Journal of Psychiatry*, 140 (3), 348–350.

Keane, T.M., & Kaloupek, D.G. (1982). Imaginal flooding in the treatment of a post-traumatic stress disorder. *Journal of Consulting and Clinical Psychology*, 550 (1), 138–140.

Keane, T. M., Zimering, R. T., & Caddell, R. T. (1985). A behavioral formulation of PTSD in Vietnam veterans. *Behavior Therapist*, 8, 9–12.

Kelly, R., & Smith, B.N. (1981). Post-traumatic syndrome: Another myth discredited. *Journal of the Royal Society of Medicine*, 74, 275–277.

Kelly, W.E. (Ed.) (1985). *Post-traumatic stress disorder and the war veteran patient*. New York: Brunner/Mazel.

Kernberg, O.F. (1975). *Borderline conditions and pathological narcissism*. New York: Jason Aronson.

Kijask, M. (1982). The syndrome of the survivor of extreme conditions. *International Review of Psychoanalysis*, 9 (1), 25–35.

Kilpatrick, D. G., Saunders, B. E., Amick-Mcmullan, A., Best, C. L., Veronen, L. J., & Resnick, H. S. (1989). Victims and crime factors associated with the development of crime-related post-traumatic stress disorder. *Behavior Therapy*, 20, 199–214 .

Kilpatrick, D. G., Veronen, L. J.,& Best, C. L. (1985). Factors predicting psychological stress amoung rape victims. In C. R. Figley (Ed.) *Trauma and its wake*. New York: Brunner/Mazel.

Kilpatrick, D. G., Saunders, B. E., Amick-McMUllan, A. Best, C. L., & Veronen, L. J. (1989). Factors affecting the development of crime-related post-traumatic stress disorder: A multivariate approach. *Behavior Therapy*.

Kilpatrick, D.G., Veronen, L.J., & Resick, P.A. (1979). The aftermath of rape: Recent empirical findings. *American Journal of Orthopsychiatry*, 49 (4), 658–669.

Kinjie, J.D. (1986). Severe posttraumatic stress disorder among Cambodian refugees: Symptoms, clinical course, and treatment approaches. In J.H. Shore (Ed.), *Disaster stress studies: New methods and findings* (123–1140). Washington, D.C.: American Psychiatric Press.

Kipper, P.A. (1977). Behavior therapy for fears brought on by war experiences. *Journal of Consulting and Clinical Psychology*, 45 (2), 216–221.

Klein, M. (1957). *Envy and gratitide: A study of unconscious sources*. New York: Basic Books.

Klonoff, H., McDougall, G., Clark, C., Kramer, P., & Hogan, J. (1979). The neuropsychological, psychiatric, and physical effects of prolonged and severe stress: 30 years later. *Journal of Nervous and Mental Disease*, 163, 246–252.

Kohut, H. (1971). *The analysis of the self*. New York: International Universities Press.

Kolb, L.C. (1977). *Modern clinical psychiatry (9th ed.)*. Philadelphia: Saunders.

Kolb, L.C. (1983). Return of the repressed: Delayed stress reaction to war. *Journal of the American Academy of Psychoanalysis*, 11 (4), 531–545.

Kolb, L. C. (1985). The place of narcosynthesis in the treatment of chronic and delayed stress reactions of war. In S.M. Sonnenberg, A. S. Blank, & J. A. Talbot (Eds.), *The trauma of war stress and recovery in Vietnam veterans*. Washington, DC: American Psychiatric Press.

Kolb, L.C., & Mutilipassi, L.R. (1982). The conditioned emotional response: A sub-class of the chronic and delayed post-traumatic stress disorder. *Psychiatric Annals*, 12 (11), 979–987.

Koocher, G. P., & O'Malley, J. E. (1981). *The Damocles syndrome*. New York: McGraw-Hill.

Kormos, H.R. (1978). The nature of combat stress. In C.R. Figley (Ed.). *Stress disorders among Vietnam veterans: Theory, research, and practice*. New York: Brunner/Mazel.

Kraft, T. (1970). A short note on 40 patients treated by systematic desensitization. *Behavioral Research and Therapy*, 8 (2), 219–220.

Krupnick, J. (1980). Brief psychotherapy with victims of violent crime. *Victimology: An International Journal*, 2–4, 347–354.

Krupnick, J.L., & Horowitz, M.J. (1981). Stress response syndromes: Recurrent themes. *Archives of General Psychiatry*, 38, 428–435.

Krystal, H. (Ed.) (1968). *Massive psychic trauma*. New York: International Universities Press.

Krystal, H. (1971a). Trauma: Considerations of its intensity and chronicity. In H. Krystal & W.G. Niederland, (Eds.), *Psychic traumatization: Aftereffects in individuals and communities*. Boston: Little, Brown.

Krystal, H. (1971b). Review of findings and implications of this symposium. In H. Krystal & W.G. Niederland (Eds.), Psychic traumatization: Aftereffects in individuals and communities. Boston: Little, Brown.

Krystal, H., & Niederland, W.G. (1968) Clinical observations on the survivor syndrome. In H. Krystal (Ed.), *Massive psychic trauma*. New York: International Universities Press.

Krystal, H., & Niederland, W.G. (1971). *Psychic traumatization: Aftereffects in individuals and communities*. Boston: Little, Brown.

Lacoursiere, R.B., Godfrey, K.E., & Ruby, L.M. (1980). Traumatic neurosis in the etiology of alcoholism: Vietnam combat and other trauma. American Journal of *Psychiatry*, 137 (8), 966–968.

Lang, P. J. (1977). The psychophysiology of anxiety. In H. Akiskal (Ed.), *Psychiatric diagnosis: Explanation of biological criteria*. New York: Spectrum.

Lankton, S., & Lankton, C. (1983). *The answer within: A clinical framework for Ericksonain hypnotherapy*. New York: Brunner/Mazel.

Lankton, S., & Lankton, C. (1987). *Enchantment and intervention*. New York: Brunner/Mazel.

Lavie, P., Hefez, A., Halpern, G., & Enoch, D. (1979). Long-term effects of traumatic war-related events on sleep. *American Journal of Psychiatry*, 136 (2), 175–178.

Lavoie, G., & Sabourin, M. (1980) Hypnosis and schizophrenia: A review of experimental and clinical studies. In *Handbook of hypnosis and psychosomatic medicine*. New York: Elsevier-North Holland.

Lazare, A., Cohen, F., Jacobson, A.M., Williams, M.W., Mignone, R.J., & Zisook, S. (1972). The walk-in patient as a "customer": A key dimension in evaluation and treatment. *American Journal of Orthopsychiatry*, 42, 872–883.

Lazarus, R., & Lavnier, R. (1978) Stress related transactions between person and environment. In L. Pervin & M. Lewis (Eds.), *Perspectives in interactional psychology.* New York:: Plenum.

Leahy, M.R., & Martin, K.A. (1963). Successful hypnotic abreaction after 20 years. *British Journal of Psychiatry*, 8, 323–333.

Leopold, R.L., & Dillon, H. (1963). Psychoanatomy of a disaster: Long-term study of post-traumatic neuroses in survivors of a marine explosion. *American Journal of Psychiatry*, 119, 913–921.

Leventman, S., & Comacho, P. (1974). The gook syndrome: The Vietnam war as a racial encounter. Paper presented at the annual meeting of the American Sociological Association, Montreal.

Levis, D.J., & Boyd, T.L. (1979). Symptom maintainance: An infrahuman analysis and extension of the conservation of anxiety principle. *Journal of Abnormal Psychology*, 88 (2), 107–120.

Levis, D.J., & Hare, N.A. (1977). Review of the theoretical rationale and empirical support for the extinction approach of implosive (flooding) therapy. In M. Hersen, R.M. Eisler, & P.M. Miller (Eds.), *Progress in behavior modification* New York: Academic Press.

Lewis, C. N. (1980). Memory adaptation to psychological trauma. *American Journal of Psychoanalysis*, 40, 319–323.

Lifton, R.J. (1967). *Death in life: Survivors of Hiroshima.* New York: Basic Books.

Lifton, R.J. (1968). *Death in life: Survivors of Hiroshima.* New York: Random House.

Lifton, R.J. (1970). The scars of Vietnam. *Commonwealth*, 91, 554–556.

Lifton, R.J. (1973). *Home from the war.* New York: Simon & Schuster.

Lifton, R. J. (1976). *The life of the self.* New York: Simon & Schuster.

Lifton, R. J. (1979). *The broken connection.* New York: Simon & Schuster.

Lifton, R.J. (1982). The psychology of the survivor and the death imprint. *Psychiatric Annals*, 12 (11), 1011–1020.

Lifton, R.J., & Olson, E. (1976). The human meaning of total disaster: The Buffalo Creek experience. *Psychiatry*, 39, 1–18.

Lindemann, E. (1944). Symptomatology and management of acute grief. *American Journal of Psychiatry*, 101 (2), 141–148.

Lindy, J.D. (1983). Vietnam veterans: A psychoanalytic study of consequences of trauma, and effects of time-limited treatment. Research in progress presentation. Annual Meeting American Psychoanalytic Association.

Lindy, J.D., & Titchener, J. (1983). "Acts of God and man": Long-term character change in survivors of disasters and the law. *Behavioral Sciences and the Law*, 1 (3), 85–96.

Lister, E. D. (1982). Forced silence: A neglected dimension of trauma. *American Journal of Psychiatry*, 139, 872–876.

Little, J.C., & Jones, B. (1964). Abreaction of a conditioned fear reaction after 18 years. *Behavioral Research and Therapy*, 2, 59–63.

Lorenzer, A. (1968). Some observations on the latency of symptoms in patients suffering from persecution sequelae. *International Journal of Psychoanalysis*, 49, 316–378.

Luchterhand, E.G. (1971). Sociological approaches to massive stress in natural and man-made disasters. In H. Krystal & W.G. Niederland (Eds.), *Psychic traumatization.* Boston: Little, Brown.

MacHovec, F.J. (1985). Treatment variables and the use of hypnosis in the brief therapy of post-traumatic stress disorders. *International Journal of Clinical and Experimental Hypnosis*, 33 (1), 6–14.

MacKenzie, T.B. (1980) Stress response syndrome occurring after delirium. *American Journal of Psychiatry*, 137 (11), 1433–1435.

Maier, S.F., & Seligman, M.E.P. (1976). Learned helplessness: Theory and evidence. *Journal of Experimental Psychology (General)*, 105, 3–46.

Malloy, P. F., Fairbank, J, A., & Keane, T. M. (1983). Validation of a multi-method assessment of post-traumatic stress disorder in Vietnam veterans. *Journal of Consulting and Clinical Psychology*, *51*, 488–494.

Malmquist, C. P. (1986). Children who witness parental murder: Posttraumatic aspects. *Journal of the American Academy of Child Psychiatry*, 25, (3), 320–325.

Mangelsdorff, A. D. (1985). Lessons learned and forgotten: The need for prevention and mental health interventions in disaster preparedness. *Journal of Community Psychology*, 13, 239–256.

Marafiote, R. (1980). Behavioral group treatment of Vietnam veterans. In T.Williams (Ed.). *Post-traumatic stress disorders of the Vietnam veteran*. Cincinnati, OH: Disabled American Veterans.

Masson, J. M. (1984) *The assault on truth: Freud's suppression of the seduction theory*. New York: Farrar, Straus & Giroux.

Masterson, J.F. (1976). *Psychotherapy for the borderline adult: A developmental approach*. New York: Brunner/Mazel.

Masterson, J.F., & Rinsley, D.B. (1975). The borderline syndrome: The role of the mother in the genesis and psychic structure of the borderline personality. *International Journal of Psychoanalysis*, 56, 163–177.

Marrs, R. (1985). Why the pain won't stop and what the family can do to help. In W.E. Kelly (Ed.), *Post-traumatic stress disorder and the war veteran patient* (885–101). New York: Brunner/Mazel.

Maruyama, M. (1963). The second cybernetics: Deviation-amplifying mutual cause processes. *American Scientist*, 51, 164–179.

McCaffrey, R.J., & Fairbank, J.A. (1985). Behavioral assessment and treatment of accident-related posttraumatic stress disorder: Two case studies. *Behavior Therapy*, 16, 406–416.

McCombe, S.L., Bassuk, E., Savitz, R., & Pell, S. (1976). Development of a medical center rape crisis intervention program. *American Journal of Psychiatry*, 133 (4), 418–421.

McCoy, A.W. (1972). *The politics of heroin in South-East Asia*. New York:Harper & Row.

McCubbin, H., & Figley, C. R. (1983). Family transitions: Adaptation to stress. In H. McCubbin & C. R. Figley (Eds.), *Stress and the family* (Vol. 1): *Coping with normative transitions*. New York: Brunner/Mazel .

McFarlane, A.C. (1986). Posttraumatic morbidity of a disaster: A study of cases presenting problems for psychiatric treatment. *Journal of Nervous and Mental Diseases*, 174 (1), 4–13.

McMahon, E. (1986). Creative self-mothering. In B. Zilbergeld, M. G. Edelstein, & D. L. Araoz (Eds.), *Hypnosis questions and answers*. New York: Norton.

Meichenbaum, D. A. (1975). A self-instructional approach to stress management: A proposal for stress inoculation training. In C. Spielberger & I. Sarason (Eds.), *Stress and anxiety* (Vol. 2). New York: Wiley.

Meichenbaum,D., & Jaremko, M. (Eds.). (1983). *Stress reduction and prevention*. New York: Plenum.

Meichenbaum, D., & Cameron, R. (1983). Stress Inoculation training: Toward a general paradigm for training in coping skills in D. Meichenbaum & M. Jaremko (Eds.), *Stress Reduction and Prevention*. New York: Plenum.

Metzger, D. (1976). It is always the woman who is raped. *American Journal of Psychiatry*, 133 (4), 405–408.

Milgram, N.A. (Ed.) (1986). *Stress and coping in time of war: Generalizations from the Israeli experience.* New York: Brunner/Mazel.

Miller, W.R., & DiPilato, M. (1983). Treatment of nightmares via relaxation and desensitization: A controlled evaluation. *Journal of Clinical and Consulting Psychology,* 51 (6), 870–877.

Minuchin, S. (1974). *Families and family therapy.* Cambridge, MA: Harvard University Press.

Moor, M. (1945). Recurrent nightmares: A simple procedure for psychotherapy. *Military Surgery,* 97, 282–285.

Musser, M.J., & Stenger, C.A. (1972). A medical and social perception of the Vietnam veteran. *Bulletin of the New York Academy of Medicine,* 48, 859–869.

Mutter, C. B. (1987). Post-traumatic stress disorder: Hypnotherapeutic approach in a most unusual case. *American Journal of Clinical Hypnosis,* 30, 81–86.

Nadelson, C.C., Notman, M.T., Zackson, H., & Gornick, J. (1982). A follow-up study of rape victims. *American Journal of Psychiatry,* 139 (10), 1266–1270.

Naples, M. (1978). The amytal interview: History and current uses. *Psychosomatics,* 19 (2), 103–105.

Newman, C.J. (1976). Children of disaster: Clinical observations at Buffalo Creek. *American Journal of Psychiatry,* 133 (3), 306–312.

Newman, L. (1979). Emotional disturbance in children of holocaust survivors. *Social Casework,* 60 (1), 43–50.

Niederland, W.G. (1968). Clinical observations on the survivor syndrome. *International Journal of Psychoanalysis,* 49 (2–3), 313–315.

Niederland, W.G. (1981). The survivor syndrome: Further observations and dimensions. *Journal of the American Psychoanalytic Association,* 29 (2), 413–425.

Niederland, W.G. (1982). Psychiatric status of a holocaust survivor (letter). *American Journal of Psychiatry,* 139 (12), 1646–1647.

Nir, Y. (1985). Post-traumatic stress disorder in children with cancer. In S. Eth & R. Pynoos (Eds.), *Post-traumatic stress disorder in children.* Washington, D. C.: American Psychiatric Press.

Norris, J., & Feldman-Summers, S. (1981). Factors related to the psychological impacts of rape on the victim. *Journal of Abnormal Psychology,* 90 (6), 562–567.

Notman, M.T., & Nadelson, C.C. (1976). The rape victim: Psychodynamic considerations. *American Journal of Psychiatry,* 133 (4), 408–413.

Novaco, R. W. (1977). Stress inoculation training: A cognitive therapy for anger and its application to a case of depression. *Journal of Consulting and Clinical Psychology,* 45 (4), 600–608.

Ochberg, F. (Ed.). (1988). *Post-traumatic therapy and victims of Violence.* New York: Brunner/Mazel.

Orne, M. T. (1969). Demand characteristics and the concept of quasi-controls. In R. Rosenthal & R. L. Rosnow (Eds.), *Artifacts in behavioral research.* New York: Academic Press.

Oswald, P., & Bittner, E. (1968). Life adjustment after severe persecution. *American Journal of Psychiatry,* 124, 1393–1400.

Panzarella, R.F., Mantell, D.M., & Bridenbaugh, R.H. (1978). Psychiatric syndromes, self-concepts, and Vietnam veterans. In C.R. Figley (Ed.), *Stress disorders among Vietnam veterans: Theory, research, and treatment* (pp. 148–172). New York: Brunner/Mazel.

Pary, R., Tobias, C., & Lippman, S. (1987). Recognizing shammed and genuine post-traumatic stress disorder. *VA Practitioner,* July, 37–43.

Penk, W.E., Robinowitz, R., Patterson, E.T., Dolan, M.P., & Atkins, H.G. (1981). Adjustment differences among male substance abusers varying in degree of combat experiences in Vietnam. *Journal of Consulting and Clinical Psychology,* 49, 426–437.

Pepitone, R.F. (1978). Patterns of rape and approaches to care. *Journal of Family Practice,* 6 (3), 521–529.

Perry, J.C., & Jacobs, D. (1982). Overview: Clinical application of the amytal interview in psychiatric emergency settings. *American Journal of Psychiatry,* 139 (5), 552–559.

Petti, T.A., & Wells, K. (1980). Crisis treatment of a preadolescent who accidentally killed his twin. *American Journal of Psychotherapy,* 34 (3), 434–443.

Pettinati, H. M. (1982). Measuring hypnotizability in psychotic patients. *International Journal of Clinical and Experimental Hypnosis,30,* 404–416.

Pilisuk, M. (1975). The legacy of the Vietnam veteran. *Journal of Social Issues,* 31 (4), 3–12.

Pynoos, R. S., & Eth, S. (1986) Witness to violence: The child interview. *Journal of the American Academy of Child Psychiatry,* 25, 306–319.

Quarentelli, E. L. (1985). An assessment of conflicting views on mental health: The consequences of traumatic events. In C. R. Figley (Ed.), *Trauma and its wake: The study and treatment of post-traumatic stress disorder.* New York: Brunner/Mazel.

Rachman, S. J. (1978). *Fear and courage.* San Francisco: W. H. Freeman.

Racker, H. (1957). The meanings and uses of countertransference. *Psychoanalytic Quarterly,* 26 (3), 303–357.

Rangell, L. (1976). Discussion of the Buffalo Creek disaster: The course of psychic trauma. *American Journal of Psychiatry,* 133 (3), 313–316.

Rappaport, E.A. (1968). Beyond traumatic neurosis: A psychoanalytic study of late reaction to the concentration camp trauma. *International Journal of Psychoanalysis,* 49, 719–730.

Reiff, R., & Scheerer, M. (1959). *Memory and hypnotic age regression.* New York: International Universities Press.

Rinsley, D.B. (1978). Borderline psychopathology: A review of aetiology, dynamics, and treatment. *International Review of Psychoanalysis,* 5, 45–54.

Rinsley, D.B. (1982). *Borderline and other self disorders: A developmental and object-relations perspective.* New York: Jason Aronson.

Roberts, W.R., Penk, W.E., Gearing, M.L., Robinowitz, R., Dolan, M.P., & Patterson, E.T. (1982). Interpersonal problems of Vietnam combat veterans with symptoms of post-traumatic stress disorder. *Journal of Abnormal Psychology,* 91 (6), 444–450.

Roth, W. T. (1988). The role of medication in post-traumatic therapy. In F. Ochberg (Ed.), *Post-traumatic therapy and victims of violence.* New York: Brunner/Mazel.

Rustin, S.L. (1972). Psychotherapy with the adolescent children of concentration camp survivors. *Journal of Contemporary Psychotherapy,* 4 (2), 87–94.

Sack, W. H., Angell, R. H., Kinzie D. & Rath, B. (1986). The psychiatric effects of massive trauma on Cambodian children: II. The family, the home, and the school. *Journal of the American Academy of Child Psychiatry,* 25, (3), 377–383.

Sank, L.I. (1979). Community disasters: Primary prevention and treatment in a health maintenance organization. *American Psychologist,* 34 (4), 334–338.

Santoli, A. (1982). *Everything we had.* New York: Ballantine.

Satir, V. (1972). *Peoplemaking.* Palo Alto, CA: Science and Behavior Books.

Saul, L. Howard, R., & Lenser, E. (1946). Desensitization of combat patients. *American Journal of Psychiatry,* 102, 476–478.

Sax, W.P. (1985). Establishing a post-traumatic stress disorder inpatient program. In W.E. Kelly (Ed.), *Post-traumatic stress disorder and the war veteran patient* (pp. 234–248). New York: Brunner/Mazel.

Schilder, F.E. (1980). Treatment by systematic desensitization of a recurring nightmare of a real life trauma. *Journal of Behavior Therapy and Experimental Psychiatry,* 11, 53–54.

Schuker, E. (1979). Psychodynamics and treatment of sex assault victims. *Journal of the American Academy of Psychoanalysis,* 7 (4), 553–573.

Scurfield, R. M. (1985). Post-trauma stress assessment and treatment: Overview and formulations. In C. R. Figley (Ed.), *Trauma and its wake: The study and treatment of posttraumatic stress disorder.* New York: Brunner/Mazel.

Seligman, M.E.P., & Maier, S.F. (1967). Failure to escape from traumatic shock. *Journal of Experimental Psychology, 74* (1), 1–9.

Seligman, M.E.P., Maier, S.F., & Geer, J. (1968). The alleviation of learned helplessness in the dog. *Journal of Abnormal Psychology, 73,* 256–262.

Shapiro, D. (1965). *Neurotic styles.* New York: Basic Books.

Shatan, C.F. (1973). The grief of soldiers: Vietnam combat veterans' self-help movement. *American Journal of Orthopsychiatry, 43* (4), 640–653.

Shatan, C.F. (1978). Stress disorder among Vietnam veterans: The emotional content of combat continues. In C.R. Figley (Ed.), *Stress disorders among Vietnam veterans: Theory, research, and practice* (pp. 43–55). New York: Brunner/Mazel.

Shatan, C.F. (1982). The tattered ego of survivors. *Psychiatric Annals, 12* (11), 1031–1038.

Shatan, C.F. (1985). Have you hugged a Vietnam veteran today? The basic wound of catastrophic stress. In W.E. Kelley (Ed.) *Post-traumatic stress disorder and the war veteran patient* (pp. 12–28). New York: Brunner/Mazel.

Sharkey, C., & Himle, D.P. (1974). Systematic desensitization of a recurring nightmare and related insomnia. *Journal of Behavior Therapy and Experimental Psychiatry, 5,* 97–98.

Shore, J.H. (Ed.). (1986). *Disaster stress studies: New methods and findings.* Washington, D.C.: American Psychiatric Press.

Sierles, F.S., Chen, J-J., Messing, M.L., Besyner, J.K., & Taylor, M.A. (1986). Concurrent psychiatric illness in non-Hispanic outpatients diagnosed as having posttraumatic stress disorder. *Journal of Nervous and Mental Disease, 174* (3), 171–173.

Silver. R.L, and Wortman, C. B. (1980). Coping with undesirable life events. In J. Garber & M.E.P. Seligman (Eds.), *Human helplessness: Theory and applications.* New York: Academic Press.

Silver, S.M. (1982). Post-traumatic stress disorders in Vietnam veterans. *Professional Psychology, 13* (4), 522–525.

Silver, S.M. (1985). Post-traumatic stress disorder and the death imprint: The search for a new mythos. In W.E. Kelly (Ed.), *Post-traumatic stress disorder and the war veteran patient* (pp. 43–53). New York: Brunner/Mazel.

Silver, S. & Iacono, C. (1984). Factor-analytic support for DSM-III's post-traumatic stress disorder for Vietnam veterans. *Journal of Clinical Psychology, 40.* 5–14.

Silver, S.M., & Kelly, W.E. (1985). Hypnotherapy of post-traumatic stress disorder in combat veterans from WW II and Vietnam. In W.E. Kelly (Ed.), *Post-traumatic stress disorder and the war veteran patient* (pp. 43–53). New York: Brunner/Mazel.

Singer, M.T. (1981). Vietnam prisoners of war, stress, and personality resiliency. *American Journal of Psychiatry, 138* (3), 345–346.

Smith, J.R. (1982). Personal responsibility in traumatic stress reactions. *Psychiatric Annals, 12* (11), 1021–1030.

Smith, J.R. (1985a). Individual psychotherapy with Viet Nam veterans. In S.M. Sonnenburg, A.S. Blank, & J.A. Talbott (Eds.), *The trauma of war: Stress and recovery in Viet Nam veterans* (pp. 125–164). Washington, DC: American Psychiatric Press.

Smith, J.R. (1985b). Rap groups and group therapy for Viet Nam veterans. In S.M. Sonnenburg, A.S. Blank, & J.A. Talbott (Eds.), *The trauma of war: Stress and recovery in Viet Nam veterans* (pp. 165–192). Washington, DC: American Psychiatric Press.

Smith, L. (1983, October). Diagnostic assessment of post-traumatic stress disorder. Workshop presented at the Second National Conference on the Treatment of Post-traumatic Stress Disorder, Chicago, IL.

Smith, S.M. (1983). Disaster: Family disruption in the wake of natural disaster. In C.R.

Figley & H.I. McCubbin (Eds.), *Stress and the family volume II: Coping with catastrophe* (pp.120–165). New York: Brunner/Mazel.

Soloman, G.F., Zarcone, V.P., Yoerg, R., Scott, N.R., & Mourer, R.G. (1971). Three psychiatric casualities from Vietnam. *Archives of General Psychiatry*, 25, 522–524.

Sonnenberg, S. M. Blank, A. S. Talbot, J. A. (Eds.). (1985). *The trauma of war stress and recovery in Vietnam veterans.* Washington, DC: American Psychiatric Press.

Sparr, L., & Pankratz, L. D. (1983). Factitious post-traumatic stress disorder. *American Journal of Psychiatry, 140,* 1016–1019.

Spiegel, D. (1981). Vietnam grief work using hypnosis. *American Journal of Clinical Hypnosis,* 24 (1), 33–40.

Spiegel, D., Hunt, T., and Dondershine, H.E. (1988). Dissociation and hypnotizability in posttraumatic stress disorder. *American Journal of Psychiatry*, 145:3, 301–305.

Spiegel, D., Detrick, D., & Frischolz, E. (1982). *American Journal of Psychiatry, 139,* 431–437.

Spiegel, D., & Spiegel, H. (1987). *Trance and treatment: Clinical uses of hypnosis.* Washington, DC: American Psychiatric Press.

Stampfl, T.G., &, Levis, D.J. (1967). Essentials of implosive therapy: A learning-based psychodynamic behavioral therapy. *Journal of Abnormal Psychology*, 72, 157–163.

Stanton, M.D., & Figley, C.R. (1978). Treating the Vietnam veteran within the family system. In C.R. Figley (Ed.), *Stress disorders among Vietnam veterans: Theory, research, and treatment* (pp. 281–290). New York: Brunner/Mazel.

Steiner, M. (1978). Traumatic neurosis and social support in the Yom Kipper war returnees. *Military Medicine*, 143 (12), 866–868.

Stern, G.M. (1976). From chaos to responsibility. *American Journal of Psychiatry*, 113 (3), 300–301.

Strange, R.E. & Brown, D.E. (1970). Home from the war: A study of psychiatric problems in Viet Nam returnees. *American Journal of Psychiatry*, 127, 130–134.

Stretch, R.H. (1985). Posttraumatic stress disorder among U.S. army reserve Vietnam and Vietnam-era veterans. *Journal of Consulting and Clinical Psychology*, 53 (6), 935–936.

Stretch, R.H., Vail, J.D., & Maloney, J.P. (1985). Posttraumatic stress disorder among army nurse corps Vietnam veterans. *Journal of Consulting and Clinical Psychology*, 53 (4), 704–708.

Stutman, R. K., Bliss,E. L. (1985). Post-traumatic stress disorder, hypnotizability, and imagery. *American Journal of Psychiatry, 142,* 741–743.

Sudak, H.S., Corradi, R.B., Martin, R.S., & Gold, F.S. (1984). Antecedent personality factors and the post-Vietnam syndrome: Case reports. *Military Medicine,* 149 (10), 550–554.

Sutherland, S., & Scherl, D.J. (1970). Patterns of response among victims of rape. *American Journal of Orthopsychiatry*, 40 (3), 503–511.

Talbott, J.A. (1982). Crisis intervention and psychoanalysis: Compatible or antagonistic? *International Journal of Psychoanalytic Psychotherapy*, 13 (2), 189–201.

Terr, L. (1979). Children of chowchilla: A study of psychic trauma. *Psychoanalytic Study of the Child, 34,* 547–623.

Terr, L.C. (1981). Forbidden games: Post-traumatic play. Journal of the *American Academy of Child Psychiatry,* 20 (4), 741–760.

Terr, L.C. (1983a). Chowchilla revisited: The effects of psychic trauma: Four years after a school-bus kidnapping. *American Journal of Psychiatry*, 140 (12), 1543–1550.

Terr, L.C. (1983b). Time sense following psychic trauma: A clincial study of ten adults and twenty children. *American Orthopsychiatric Association*, 53 (2), 244–261.

Terr, L. (1985). Children traumatized in small groups. In S. Eth & R. Pynoos (Eds.), *Post-traumatic stress disorder in children.* Washington, D. C.: American Psychiatric Press.

Theines-Hontos, P., Watson, G.G., & Kucala, T. (1982). Stress-disorder symptoms in Vietnam and Korean war veterans. *Journal of Consulting and Clinical Psychology*, 50 (4), 588–561.

Tichener, J.L., & Kapp, F.T. (1976). Family and character change at Buffalo Creek. *American Journal of Psychiatry*, 133 (3), 295–299.

Trimble, M.R. (1981). *Post-traumatic naurosis: From railway spine to the whiplash*. Chichester, U.K.: Wiley.

Trimble, M. R. (1985). Post-traumatic stress disorder: History of a concept. In C. R. Figley (Ed.), *Trauma and its wake: The study and treatment of post-traumatic stress disorder*. New York: Brunner/Mazel.

van der Kolk, B.A. (1983). Psychopharmocological issues in posttraumatic stress disorder. *Hospital and Community Psychiatry*, *34*, 683–691.

van der Kolk, B. A. (Ed.). (1984). Posttraumatic stress disorder: Psychological and biological sequelae. Washington, D.C: American Psychiatric Press.

van der Kolk, B. A. (1988). The biological response to trauma. In F. Ochberg (Ed.), *Posttraumatic therapy and victims of violence*. New York: Brunner/Mazel.

van der Kolk, B.A., & Ducey, C. P. (1984). Clinical implications of the Rorshach in posttraumatic stress. In B. A. van der Kolk (Ed.), Posttraumatic stress disorder: Psychological and biological sequelae. Washington, D.C: American Psychiatric Press.

van der Kolk, B.A., Boyd, H., Krystal J., et al. (1984). Post-traumatic stress disorder as a biologically based disorder: Implications of the animal model of inescapable shock. In B. A. van der Kolk (Ed.) Posttraumatic stress disorder: Psychological and biological sequelae. Washington, D.C: American Psychiatric Press.

van der Kolk, B.A., Greenberg, M. S., Boyd, H., & Krystal, J (1985). Inescapable shock, neurotransmitters and addiction to trauma. Towards a psychobiology of post-traumatic stress. *Biological Psychiatry*, *20*, 314–325.

van Dyke, C., Zilberg, N.J., & McKinnon, J.A. (1985). Posttraumatic stress disorder: A thirty-year delay in a WW II veteran. *American Journal of Psychiatry*, 142 (9), 1070–1073.

van Kampen, M., Watson, C.G., Tilleskjor, C., Kucala, T., & Vassar, P. (1986). The definition of posttraumatic stress disorder in alcoholic Vietnam veterans: Are the DSM-III criteria necessary and sufficient? *Journal of Nervous and Mental Diseases*, 174 (3), 137–143.

Veronen, L. J., & Kilpatrick, D. G. (1980). Self-reported fears of rape victims: A preliminary investigation. *Behavior Modification*, 4,(3), 383–396.

Veronen, L. J. & Kilpatrick, D. G. (1983). Stress management for rape victims. In D. Meichenbaum & M. Jaremko (Eds.). *Stress reduction and prevention*. New York: Plenum.

Walker, J.I. (1981a). Vietnam veterans with legal difficulties: A psychiatric problem? *American Journal of Psychiatry*, 138 (10), 1384–1385.

Walker, J.I. (1981b). The psychological problem of the Vietnam veteran. *Journal of the American Medical Association*, 246 (7), 781–782.

Walker, J.I. (1982). Chemotherapy of traumatic war stress. *Military Medicine*, 147 (2), 1029–1033.

Walker, J.I., & Mash, J.L. (1981). Group therapy in the treatment of Vietnam combat veterans. International *Journal of Group Psychotherapy*, 31 (3), 379–389.

Watkins, J.G. (1971). The affect bridge. *International Journal of Clinical and Experimental Hypnosis*, 19, 21–27.

Watkins, J. G., & Watkins, H. H. (1981). The theory and practice of ego-state therapy. In H. Grayson (Ed.), Short-term approaches to psychotherapy. New York: Human Sciences Press.

Weakland, J.H., Fisch, R., Watzlawick, P., & Bodin, A.M. (1974). Brief family therapy: Focused problem resolution. *Family Process*, 13, 141–168.

Weitzenhoffer, A.M. (1953). *General techniques of hypnotism.* New York: Wiley.

Wilkinson, C.B. (1983). Aftermath of a disaster: The collapse of the Hyatt Regency Hotel Skywalks. *American Journal of Psychiatry,* 140 (9), 1134–1139.

Williams, C.C. (1983). The mental foxhole: The Vietnam veteran's search for meaning. *American Journal of Orthopsychiatry,* 53 (1), 4–17.

Williams, C.M. (1980). The veteran system with a focus on women partners: Theoretical considerations, problems, and treatment strategies. In T. Williams (Ed.), *Post-traumatic stress disorders of the Vietnam veteran* (pp. 73–122). Cincinnati, OH: Disabled American Veterans.

Williams, C.M., & Williams, T. (1985). Family therapy for Vietnam veterans. In S.M. Sonnenberg, A.S. Blank, & J.A. Talbott (Eds.), *The trauma of war: Stress and recovery in Vietnam veterans* (193–209). Washington, DC: American Psychiatric Press.

Williams, T. (1980a). Therapeutic alliance and goal setting in the treatment of Vietnam veterans. In T. Williams (Ed.), *Post-traumatic stress disorders of the Vietnam veteran* (pp. 25–36). Cincinnati, OH: Disabled American Veterans.

Williams, T. (1980b). A preferred model for development of interventions for psychogical readjustment of Vietnam veterans: Group treatment. In T. Williams (Ed.), *Post-traumatic stress disorders of the Vietnam veteran* (37–48). Cincinnati, OH: Disabled American Veterans.

Wilmer, H.A. (1982a). Vietnam and madness: Dreams of schizophrenic veterans. *Journal of the American Academy of Psychoanalysis,* 10 (1), 47–65.

Wilmer, H.A. (1982b). Dream seminar for chronic schizophrenic patients. *Psychiatry,* 45, 351–360.

Wilmer, H.A. (1982c). Post-traumatic stress disorder. *Psychiatric Annals,* 12 (11), 995–1003.

Wilson, A., & Fromm, E. (1982). Aftermath of the concentration camp: The second generation. *Journal of the American Academy of Psychoanalysis,* 10 (2), 289–313.

Wilson, J.P. (1977). *Identity, ideology, and crisis: The Vietnam veteran in transition* (Vol. 1). Washington D.C.: Disabled American Veterans.

Wilson, J.P. (1978). *Identity, ideology, and crisis: The Vietnam veteran in transition* (Vol. 2). Washington D.C.: Disabled American Veterans.

Wilson, J. P. (1980). Conflict, stress and growth: The effects of war on psychosocial development amoung Vietnam veterans, In C. R. Figley & S. Leventman (Eds.), Strangers at home: *Vietnam veterans since the war.* New York: Praeger.

Wilson, J.P. (Speaker). (1983). New theoretical dimensions of PTSD (cassette recording). Dayton, OH: Serco Marketing & Human Resources Initiative.

Wilson, J.P., & Krauss, G.E. (1985). Predicting post-traumatic stress disorders among Vietnam veterans. In W.E. Kelly (Ed.), *Post-traumatic stress disorder and the war veteran patient* (pp. 102–147). New York: Brunner/Mazel.

Winnik, H.Z. (1969). Contribution to symposium on psychic traumatization through social catastrophe. *International Journal of Psychoanalysis,* 49 (2–3), 298–230.

Wise, M.G. (1983). Post-traumatic stress disorder: The human reaction to catastrophe. *Drug Therapy,* 13 (3), 62–69.

Wolberg, L.R. (1945). *Hypnoanalysis.* New York: Grune & Stratton.

Worthington, E.R. (1978). Demographic and preservice variables as predictors of post-military adjustment. In C.R. Figley (Ed.), *Stress disorders among Vietnam veterans: Theory, research, and treatment* (173–187). New York: Brunner/Mazel.

Wortman, C. B., & Silver, R. C. (1987) Coping with irrecovable loss in G.R. VandenBos & B.K. Bryant (Eds.), *Cataclysm, crises and catastrophes: Psychology in Action — Master Lecture Series.* Washington, DC: American Psychological Association.

Yager, J. (1976). Postcombat violent behavior in psychiatrically maladjusting soldiers. *Archives of General Psychiatry,* 33, 1332–1335.

Yager, T., Laufer, R., & Gallops, M. (1984). Some problems associated with war experience in men of the Vietnam generation. *Archives of General Psychiatry, 41,* 327–333.

Yalom, I. D. (1975). *The theory and practice of group psychotherapy* (2nd ed.). New York: Basic Books.

Yost, J. (1980). The psychopharmacologic treatment of the delayed stress syndrome in Vietnam veterans. In T. Williams (Ed.), *Post-traumatic stress disorders of the Vietnam veteran* (pp. 125–132). Cincinnati, OH: Disabled American Veterans.

Zusman, J., & Simon, J. (1983). Difference in repeated psychiatric examinations of litigants to a lawsuit. *American Journal of Psychiatry, 140:*10, 1300–1304.

Index

PTSD refers to post-traumatic stress disorder.

Abreaction in PTSD therapy, 6
  in behavioral therapy with children,
    209–211
  in hypnotherapy, 174–175, 179
  in narcosynthesis, 181
Accidental manmade disasters, PTSD in
    survivors of, 47, 55–58
Accountability issues, in therapy of
    childhood PTSD, 207
Active role in traumatic event, assessment
    of, 124
Acute PTSD, 43–44
  therapy in, 144
Adaptive behavior, 4–5, 6
  assessment of, 126–127
  ecosystemic model of PTSD on, 103
  psychosocial model of PTSD on, 73, 74,
    75
  in rape victims, 53
  in reexperiencing of traumatic event,
    20–21
  in resolution of PTSD, 47–48, 49
Adjustment disorders, differential
    diagnosis of, 116–118
Affect, restricted range of, in PTSD, 22–
    23
Age-sounding technique, in family
    therapy for PTSD, 200
Aggressive behavior in PTSD, 28

Alcohol use in PTSD, 38–39
  assessment of, in forensic evaluation,
    130, 132
  and problems in
    psychopharmacological therapy,
    215
Alertness, increased, in PTSD, 30–31. *See
    also* Arousal symptoms of PTSD
Amnesia, psychogenic, in PTSD, 24
  hypnotherapy in, 173–174
Anger in PTSD, 28–30
  behavioral theories on, 76–77, 169
  in maladaptive resolution, 49, 50
  stress inoculation training in, 169
Antidepressant drug therapy in PTSD,
    213, 214, 215, 216
Antipsychotic drug therapy in PTSD, 216
Antisocial personality disorder,
    differential diagnosis of, 118–120
Anxiety, in PTSD, 37, 116
  of children, 63
  in death imprint, 37–38
  drug therapy in, 214–215
Anxiety disorders, differential diagnosis
    of, 116
Appraisals, cognitive, in PTSD, 53, 54,
    78–82, 97–101
  of children, 211
  on justice system, 55, 80, 101

247

Appraisals, cognitive, in PTSD (*cont.*)
  on life threats, 54, 80, 101
Arousal symptoms of PTSD, 26–31, 93,
      94, 99
  drug therapy in, 94, 214–215
  heart rate in, 26, 27, 30
  hyperalertness and hypervigilance in,
      30–31
  anger, rage, and hostility in, 28–30
  memory and concentration in, 27–28
  in reexperiencing of traumatic event,
      30
  sleep difficulties in, 27
Assertiveness training in PTSD, 186
Assessment of PTSD, 105–139
  adverse interactional styles affecting,
      135
  attitude of examiner affecting, 134
  on attributions of meaning, 126
  behavioral procedures in, 114
  bias of examiner in, 123, 133, 138
  comorbidity theory on, 138
  on coping responses, 124–125
  corroboration of data in, 135–136
  differential diagnosis in, 115–123
  DSM-III criteria in, 108–115, 134–135
  exaggeration and falsification of data
      in, 136–137
    differential diagnosis of, 120–123
  in family therapy, 199
  in forensic situations, 121, 122–123,
      127–133. *See also* Forensic
      assessment of PTSD
  functional evaluation in, 123–127
  future changes in, 9, 220
  history of patient in, 123–124, 130, 131–
      132
  impact of examiner in, 123, 127, 133–
      135, 138
  impact on examiner, 138–139
  on intercurrent stressors, 137
  interview technique in, 109, 110–111,
      122, 136
  mental status examination in, 111
  Minnesota Multiphasic Personality
      Inventory in, 112–114, 121, 220
  in multiple disorders, 137–138
  problems in, 133–139
  in psychodynamic approach, 152–154
  psychometric and psychodiagnostic
      testing in, 111–115

Assessment of PTSD (*cont.*)
  on psychosocial context
    post-trauma, 125–126
    pre-trauma, 124
  screening in, 108, 109
  self-report inventories in, 115
  in silent or reluctant patients, 122, 136
  on strengths and resources of patient,
      126–127
Atomic explosions in Japan, PTSD in
      survivors of, 58–59. *See also*
      Hiroshima and Nagasaki survivors,
      PTSD in Attributions of meaning
      in PTSD, 5, 6
  alteration of, in therapy, 145, 146, 148
  assessment of, 126
  of rape victims, 53
Avoidance behavior in PTSD, 5, 12–14,
      25–26, 99
  behavioral theory on, 77
  of children, 63
  diagnostic criteria on, 12–14
  ecosystemic model on, 97
  therapy decreasing, 145, 146, 147

Beck Depression Inventory, 115
Behavioral theories on PTSD, 75–78,
      159–160
  in assessment procedure, 114
  in biological model, 93, 94
  in cybernetic model, 94, 95
  historical, 5
  in therapy, 7, 146, 159–169
    of children, 209–211
    desensitization in, systematic, 7, 145,
        163–164, 211
    effectiveness of, 162–163, 164, 169
    in groups, 184, 184–187
    implosive (imaginal flooding)
        procedure in, 145, 160–163
    rehearsal in, 7, 145, 164–165, 186
    stress inoculation training in, 7, 145,
        165–169, 205, 211, 219
Benzodiazepine therapy in PTSD, 213,
      215
Bereavement, differential diagnosis of
      adjustment disorder and PTSD in,
      117
Bias of mental health professionals, in
      assessment and diagnosis of PTSD,
      123, 133, 138

Biological model of PTSD, 91–94
  arousal symptoms in, 31, 93, 214
  drug therapy in, 94, 214
Blaming of self in PTSD
  in rape victims, 53
  and survivor guilt, 33
Blood pressure, and increased arousal in
    PTSD, 26
Borderline personality disorder, 120
Brain activity in PTSD, in
    psychophysiologic and
    psychobiologic models, 92, 93, 214
Buffalo Creek disaster survivors, PTSD
    in, 41
  assessment of, 122–123
  in children, 61
  course of, 55, 56, 57
  death imprint in, 38

Cambodian refugees, PTSD in, 17
  anger, irritability, and violence as
    symptoms of, 29
  in children, 62, 63, 64, 65
  detachment and estrangement feelings
    in, 23
  distress in reexperiencing trauma in, 20
  nightmares in, 18
  startle response in, 30
Cancer in children, and PTSD, 63, 64
  parental response affecting, 64
Central nervous system activity in PTSD,
    psychophysiologic and
    psychobiologic models on, 92, 93,
    94, 214
Children, PTSD in, 61–66
  diagnostic criteria on, 14
  diminished interest in activities in, 14,
    22
  dreams and nightmares in, 14, 63, 208
  grief in, 211
  guilt feelings in, 32
  occurrence of, 61–62
  parental response to, 64–65
  revenge fantasies in, 207, 209, 211, 212
  self-image in, 63, 208, 212
  symptoms of, 14, 62–63
  in terrorist attacks, 24, 32
  therapy of, 205–212
    behavioral approach in, 168–169,
      209–211
    closure stage in, 208–209

Children, PTSD in (cont.)
  therapy of (cont.)
    in groups, 205, 209, 210, 211
    interview technique in, 205–209
    opening stage of, 205–206
    reconstruction and coping with
      trauma in, 206–208
    stress inoculation training in, 168–
      169, 205, 211
  time sense alterations in, 14, 24, 40, 62
Chowchilla, PTSD in children from, 62,
    65
Chronic PTSD, 44
  conditioned emotional response in, 45
  delayed, 44–45
  therapy in, 144
Clonidine therapy in PTSD, 213, 214
Cognitive functioning in PTSD, 5–6
  appraisals in. See Appraisals, cognitive,
    in PTSD
  attributions of meaning in, 5, 6, 126,
    145, 146, 148
  ecosystemic model on, 96, 97, 101
  information-processing model on, 70
  memory and concentration in, 27–28
  in therapy, 7
    of children, 211
    in group approach, 184, 185–187
Combat-related PTSD, 8, 18
  and antisocial personality disorder, 118–
    119
  course of, 51
  disability payments in, 121, 122
  dreams and nightmares in, 17, 18, 190–
    191
  factitious, 121, 122, 136
  flashbacks in, 18, 19
  historical aspects of, 3, 4, 5, 6–7
  irritability, anger, and rage in, 28–29
  learned repression in, 25
  Minnesota Multiphasic Personality
    Inventory in assessment of, 113–
    114, 121
  narcosynthesis in, 30, 45
  paranoia in, 31
  psychoanalytic theories on, 82
  shell shock in, 3, 4
  sleep difficulties in, 27, 215
  in Vietnam veterans. See Vietnam
    veterans, PTSD in
Communication, in family therapy for
    PTSD, 195, 200, 201

Community response to PTSD,
    assessment of, 126
Comorbidity theory in diagnosis of PTSD,
    138
Compensation in PTSD, financial. *See*
    Financial compensation in PTSD
Completion tendency in PTSD,
    information-processing model on,
    70
Concentration, difficulties in, in PTSD,
    27–28
Concentration camp survivors, PTSD in
    anxiety in, 37
    arousal symptoms in, 27, 31
    diminished interest in activities in, 22
    dissociative reactions in, 18, 19
    distress in exposure to symbolic
        representation of event in, 20
    dreams and nightmares in, 18
    family therapy in, 197–198
    personality in, 41
    psychoanalytic theories on, 83, 84
    rage in, 29
    restricted range of affect in, 22, 23
    and schizophrenia, 120
    sleep difficulties in, 27
    somatic symptoms of, 39
Conditioning
    and arousal symptoms of PTSD, 31
    behavioral theory of PTSD on, 76–77
    ecosystemic model of PTSD on, 97
    and emotional responses in PTSD, 30,
        45
Conduct disturbances in PTSD of
    children, 63
Constructivism, 6
Contracts, in group therapy for PTSD,
    185, 187
Control systems in PTSD therapy
    in children, 207–208
    in hypnotherapy, 172–173
    in psychodynamic therapy, 153, 154
Coping skills in PTSD
    in adaptive resolution, 21
    assessment of, 124–125, 130
    of children, 64, 207–208
    cognitive appraisal model on, 78, 101
    ecosystemic model on, 101
    psychosocial model on, 72, 73, 74
    therapy supporting, 144, 145, 146
        in children, 207–208

Coping skills in PTSD (*cont.*)
    therapy supporting (*cont.*)
    in family therapy, 195
    in hypnotherapy, 177
    in stress inoculation training, 166,
        168
Corroboration of data, in assessment of
    PTSD, 135–136
Countertransference phenomena in group
    therapy for PTSD, 184, 187, 188,
        189
Couples in PTSD therapy, 7, 203
Course of PTSD, 45–60
    in accidental manmade disasters, 47,
        55–58
    in Buffalo Creek disaster survivors, 55,
        56, 57
    in combat veterans, 51
    ecosystemic model on, 103
    in Hiroshima survivors, 58–59
    information-processing model on, 71
    phases in, 46, 152
    possible trajectories in, 47–49
    in rape victims, 51–55
    stage theory on, 46–47
    in Three Mile Island residents, 59
Crime victims, PTSD in
    concentration in, 28
    course of, 51–55
    depression in, 36, 37
    dreams and nightmares in, 18
    guilt feelings in, 32, 33
    intrusive symptoms in, 17
    rage in, 29
    in rape. *See* Rape victims, PTSD in
Crisis theory, 143–144, 219
Cues, in behavioral theory of PTSD, 76
    in implosive therapy, 161–162
Cultural factors in PTSD, 7–8
    assessment of, 126
    behavioral theory on, 77
Cybernetic model of PTSD, 94–96, 102
    cybernetic deviation amplification
        circuit in, 94, 102–103

Damocles syndrome in cancer and PTSD
    of children, 63
Death, PTSD associated with, 9, 37–38,
    218
    and bereavement as normal
        developmental experience, 117

Death, PTSD associated with (*cont.*)
  and cognitive appraisal of life-
    threatening events, 54, 80, 101
  and ghosts reported by children, 63
  imprint and anxiety in, 37–38
  in Hiroshima survivors, 58
  in rape victims, 54
Defendant, forensic evaluation of PTSD
    for
  agenda of, 130, 131–132
  ethical issues in, 127–128, 129
  interpretations and conclusions in, 132–
    133
Defensive behavior in PTSD
  ecosystemic model on, 101
  information-processing model on, 70,
    71
  psychodynamic therapy in, 152–153
  psychosocial model on, 72, 73, 74
Delayed PTSD, 44
  chronic, 44–45
  conditioned emotional response in, 45
  therapy in, 144
Denial phase of PTSD, 46
  in children, 62, 63
  information-processing model on, 70,
    71
  therapy in, 146
    family approach to, 199
    psychodynamic, 152, 154, 155
Depression in PTSD, 36–37
  assessment of, 115, 116
  drug therapy in, 215
  substance abuse in, 38, 39
Descriptions of PTSD, historical, 3–4
Desensitization, systematic, in behavioral
    therapy of PTSD, 7, 145, 163–164
  in children, 211
Detachment, feelings of, in PTSD, 23–24
  psychosocial-developmental theory on,
    85, 86
Development, psychosocial, and PTSD,
    84–86
  in psychoformative theory, 87–88
Developmental skills of children, loss of,
    in PTSD, 14, 22
Diagnosis of PTSD, 1–66
  assessment procedures in, 105–139. *See
    also* Assessment of PTSD
  characteristics of traumatic stressor in,
    15–16

Diagnosis of PTSD (*cont.*)
  and course of disorder, 45–60
  and differential diagnosis, 115–123
  DSM-III criteria in. *See* DSM-III
    criteria on PTSD
  DSM-III-R criteria in. *See* DSM-III-R
    criteria on PTSD
  future trends in, 9, 220
  historical aspects of, 3–4
  primary symptoms in, 11–34
  problems in, 133–139
  secondary symptoms in, 11, 35–42
  and subtypes of disorder, 43–45
Disability payments in PTSD, 121, 122. *See
    also* Financial compensation in
    PTSD
Disaster survivors, PTSD in, 36, 37, 47
  in Buffalo Creek residents. *See* Buffalo
    Creek disaster survivors, PTSD in
  course of, 47, 55–58
Disorganization phase of rape trauma
    syndrome, 52–53, 54
Dissociative reactions in PTSD, 18–20, 45
  hypnotherapy in, 171, 172, 173, 174,
    176, 177
  in maladaptive resolution, 49, 50
  narcosynthesis in, 45, 181
Drawing and storytelling, in therapy of
    childhood PTSD, 206
Dreams and nightmares in PTSD, 17–18
  of children, 14, 63, 208
  continuing after waking, 18, 19
  desensitization in, systematic, 163, 164
  diagnostic criteria on, 17
  drug therapy in, 215
  in Jungian approach to group therapy,
    184, 190–191
  and sleep difficulties, 27
Drug abuse in PTSD, 38–39
  assessment of, in forensic evaluation,
    130, 132
  and problems in
    psychopharmacological therapy,
    215
Drug therapy in PTSD, 213–216
  in arousal and anxiety, 94, 214–215
  cybernetic model on, 95
  in depression, 215
  indications for, 216
  in narcosynthesis, 6, 30, 45, 180–181
  in psychotic-like behavior, 216

Drug therapy in PTSD (*cont.*)
  rationales for, 213–214
  in sleep disturbances, 191, 215
  withdrawal of, 216
DSM-I, 3
DSM-II, 3
DSM-III criteria on PTSD, 4, 11, 12
  adherence to, in assessment procedure,
    134–135
  assessment of, in formal diagnostic
    procedure, 108–115
  compared to DSM-III-R criteria, 12–15
  in differential diagnosis, 116
  on subtypes of disorder, 43, 44
  on traumatic stressor, 15
DSM-III-R criteria on PTSD, 4, 9, 11, 13
  arousal symptoms in, 26
  assessment of, in formal diagnostic
    procedure, 108, 113
  avoidance behavior in, 12–14, 25
  on children, 14
  compared to DSM-III criteria, 12–15
  psychogenic amnesia in, 24
  on subtypes of disorder, 43, 44
  on traumatic stressor, 15

Earthquake survivors, PTSD in, 209, 210
Ecosystemic model of PTSD, 96–103
  diagram of, 100
Ego functioning in PTSD, 41
  historical view of, 4
  information-processing model on, 70
  psychoanalytic theories on, 83, 84
  psychosocial model on, 72, 74
  therapy supporting, 144, 145, 146, 173
Electric shock therapy, historical use of, 6
Emotional reactions in PTSD
  in children, 206
  conditioned response in, 30, 45
  detachment and estrangement in, 23–
    24
  irritability, anger, and rage in, 28–30
  numbing of responsiveness in. *See*
    Numbing of responsiveness in
    PTSD
  psychodynamic approach to, 153, 155
  in rape victims, 53
  restricted range of, 22–23
Environmental influences in PTSD
  cybernetic model on, 95

Environmental influences in PTSD (*cont.*)
  ecosystemic model on, 96, 97
  psychosocial model on, 72, 73, 74
Estrangement, feelings of, in PTSD, 23–
    24
  psychosocial-developmental theory on,
    85, 86
Ethical issues in forensic evaluation of
    PTSD, 8, 127–129
Evaluation of PTSD, 105–139. *See also*
    Assessment of PTSD
Exaggeration of data, in assessment of
    PTSD, 136–137
  differential diagnosis of, 120–123
Examiner. *See* Mental health professionals

Factitious PTSD, 120–123, 136–137
Falsification of data, in assessment of
    PTSD, 136–137
  differential diagnosis of, 120–123
Family of PTSD patient, 23
  assessment of, 125, 199–200
  characteristics of, 196–198
  of origin, 198
  of procreation, 198
  in therapy, 7, 145, 193–203
    age-sounding technique in, 200
    effectiveness of, 203
    goals of, 194–196, 201–202
    healing theory in, 201
    integration with other treatment
      modalities, 202–203
    procedures in, 194
    reframing of problem in, 200–201
    role of therapist in, 194, 200, 202
    theoretical assumptions in, 194
    ventilation phase of, 200
Fear response in PTSD
  assessment of, 115
  behavioral theory on, 76
    in desensitization therapy, 164
    in stress inoculation training, 168
  in children, 63, 207, 208
  ecosystemic model on, 97
  in maladaptive resolution, 49, 50
  in rape victims, 53
Financial compensation in PTSD, 3, 8, 9,
    218
  ethical issues in, 127–129
  and exaggeration and falsification of
    data, 120, 121, 122, 136

Financial compensation in PTSD (*cont.*)
  future trends in, 9, 218
  historical aspects of, 3
Flashbacks in PTSD, 18, 19
  in children, 62
Flooding procedure in behavioral therapy
    of PTSD, 145, 160–163
Forensic assessment of PTSD, 121, 122–
    123, 127–133
  conflicting results in, 122–123
  for defense, 127–128, 129, 130, 131–132
  ethical issues in, 8, 127–129
  exaggeration of responses in, 120–123,
    136–137
  examiner bias in, 123
  interpretations and conclusions in, 132–
    133
  negative attitudes of mental health
    professionals in, 134
  null hypothesis in, 129
  for plaintiff, 128–129, 130, 132–133
Foreshortened future sense in PTSD, 40
  in children, 14, 24, 62
Functional evaluation of PTSD, 123–127
Future, foreshortened, sense of, in PTSD,
    40
  in children, 14, 24, 62
Future trends in PTSD, 8–9, 218–221

Generalization of stimulus, in behavioral
    theory of PTSD, 76
Ghosts, reported in PTSD of children, 63
Grief reactions in PTSD, 23, 24
  of children, 211
  and differential diagnosis of normal
    developmental processes, 117
Group therapy in PTSD, 7, 183–192
  children in, 205, 209, 210, 211
  cognitive-behavioral approach in, 184,
    185–187
  combined with individual therapy, 191
  dream seminars in, 184, 190–191
  effectiveness of, 191–192
  hypnotherapy in, 173
  interactive, 184–185
  narcosynthesis in, 180
  psychoanalytic, 184, 187–189
  theoretical orientations in, 183–184
Guilt feelings in PTSD, 14, 31–33
  of rape victims, 53
  and self-blaming, 33

Guilt feelings in PTSD (*cont.*)
  of survivors, 14, 31–33, 59

Hallucinations in PTSD, 18, 19
Heart rate, and arousal symptoms of
    PTSD, 26, 27, 30
Helplessness, feelings of, in PTSD
  biological model on, 93
  cognitive appraisal model on, 81
  and depression, 37
  and time sense alterations, 40
Hiroshima and Nagasaki survivors, PTSD
    in
  course of, 58–59
  and schizophrenia, 120
  symptoms of, 22, 29, 32
Historical aspects of PTSD, 3–8
  in cultural and political influences, 7–8
  in description and diagnosis, 3–4
  in theories, 4–6
  in therapy, 6–7
History of patient in PTSD, 123–124
  in forensic evaluation, 130, 131–132
Hostages, PTSD in, 36, 37
Hostility in PTSD, 28–30
Hyatt Regency Hotel collapse, PTSD in
    survivors of, 17, 20, 29–30
Hyperalertness in PTSD, 30–31. *See also*
    Arousal symptoms of PTSD
Hypervigilance in PTSD, 30–31. *See also*
    Arousal symptoms of PTSD
Hypnotherapy in PTSD, 6, 7, 145, 171–
    180
  abreaction in, 174–175, 179
  effectiveness of, 179–180
  indications and contraindications to,
    178–179
  as integrative technique, 175–178, 179
  restructuring of traumatic event in, 175
  self-hypnotic techniques in, 173
  as supportive technique, 172–173, 179
  theoretical assumptions in, 171–172
  as uncovering technique, 173–174, 179
Hysterical style of information processing
    in PTSD, 71
  psychodynamic therapy in, 152, 156–
    157

Identification
  with killer, in object-relations theory on
    PTSD, 90, 176

Identification (*cont.*)
  in transference/countertransference
    phenomena, in group therapy for
    PTSD, 188
  with victim, in object-relations theory
    on PTSD, 90, 176
Identity, sense of, in PTSD. *See* Self-image
    in PTSD
Illness, adjustment disorder and PTSD in,
    117
Illusions in PTSD, 18
Imagery techniques in PTSD therapy
  in behavioral therapy, 160–163, 166
  in hypnotherapy, 173, 174, 175
Impact of Events Scale, 62, 115, 220
Impact reactions in rape trauma
    syndrome, 52
Implosive therapy, in behavioral approach
    to PTSD, 7, 160–163
Impulsive behavior in PTSD, 38
  in children, 207–208
Informative-processing in PTSD, 69–72
  historical view of, 5–6
  hysterical style of, 71, 152, 156–157
  obsessional style of, 71–72, 152, 157–
    158, 186
  psychodynamic theories on, 152, 154–
    155, 156–158
  psychophysiologic model on, 92, 94
Insurance payments in PTSD, 8, 9, 127–
    129, 218. *See also* Financial
    compensation in PTSD
Intelligence tests in PTSD, 111
Interactive group therapy in PTSD, 184–
    185
Interest in activities, diminished, in
    PTSD, 14, 22
Interview technique in PTSD
  in assessment procedures, 109, 110–111
  silence or reluctance of patient in, 122,
    136
  in therapy of childhood PTSD, 205–209
Intimate relationships in PTSD, 22, 23,
    196, 197
  psychosocial-developmental theory on,
    85, 86
Intrusive symptoms of PTSD, 16–21, 46
  adaptive value of, 20–21
  in children, 14, 62, 63
  death imprint in, 37–38

Intrusive symptoms of PTSD (*cont.*)
  dreams and nightmares in, 17–18
  drug therapy in, 214
  ego-supportive interventions in, 146
  in exposure to symbolic representation
    of trauma, 20–21
  family therapy in, 199
  hypnotherapy in, 175
  illusions, hallucinations, and flashbacks
    in, 18–20
  information-processing model on, 70, 71
  in oscillation phase, 46, 49
  psychodynamic therapy in, 152, 154,
    155, 156
Irritability in PTSD, 28–30
Isolation, feelings of, in PTSD, 23–24, 196
  psychosocial-developmental theory on,
    85, 86

Japan, PTSD in Hiroshima and Nagasaki
    survivors. *See* Hiroshima and
    Nagasaki survivors, PTSD in
Jungian dream seminars in group therapy
    for PTSD, 184, 190–191
Justice system, victim satisfaction with,
    and PTSD, 55, 80, 101

Killer-self, in object relations theory on
    PTSD, 90, 176

Learning theory on PTSD, 5, 75–78
  arousal symptoms in, 31
  in group therapy, 184, 185–187
  repression in, 25
Legal issues in PTSD, 8, 9
  in assessment procedures. *See* Forensic
    assessment of PTSD
Life threatening events, PTSD in
  cognitive appraisal model on, 54, 80,
    101
  death imprint and death anxiety in,
    37–38, 54, 58
Lithium therapy in PTSD, 213, 214

Maladaptive resolution of PTSD, 48–49
  beliefs and symptoms in, 50
  cognitive appraisal model on, 78
Malingering, 4, 120–123
Memory in PTSD
  behavioral theory on, 77, 159, 161
  cybernetic model on, 94, 95

Memory in PTSD (*cont.*)
  and hypnotherapy as uncovering
    technique, 173–174
  impairment of, 27–28
  and psychogenic amnesia, 24, 173–174
  recurrent or distressing recollections in,
    16–17
Mental health professionals
  affecting assessment of PTSD, 123, 127,
    133–135, 138
    in adherence to DSM-III criteria,
      134–135
    in bias, 123, 133, 138
    in negative attitudes, 134
  assessment procedure affecting, 138–
    139
  expectations of, affecting course of
    PTSD, 24
  role of, in therapy
    in ego-supportive interventions, 146
    in family therapy, 194, 200, 202
    in group therapy, 184–185
    in hypnotherapy, 172, 173, 174, 178
    recurring problems related to, 149
Mental status examination in PTSD, 111
  in forensic evaluation, 130
Military combat, PTSD related to. *See*
  Combat-related PTSD
Minnesota Multiphasic Personality
  Inventory (MMPI), in assessment of
  PTSD, 112–114, 121, 220
Modeling techniques in PTSD therapy,
  186
Monamine oxidase inhibitor therapy in
  PTSD, 213, 215
Mourning reactions in PTSD, 23, 24
  of children, 211
  and differential diagnosis of normal
    developmental processes, 117

Nagasaki survivors, PTSD in. *See*
  Hiroshima and Nagasaki survivors,
  PTSD in
Narcosynthesis in PTSD therapy, 6, 30,
  45, 180–181
Neurologic factors in PTSD
  historical view of, 4
  psychophysiologic and psychobiologic
    models on, 92, 93, 94, 214
Neurosis
  compensation, 3

Neurosis (*cont.*)
  traumatic, 3, 56
Nightmares in PTSD. *See* Dreams and
  nightmares in PTSD
Nuclear accident at Three Mile Island,
  and PTSD, 28, 59, 65
Null hypothesis in forensic evaluation of
  PTSD, 129
Numbing of responsiveness in PTSD, 12,
  21–25, 46, 99, 146
  avoidance behaviors in, 25–26
  behavioral theory on, 77
  in Buffalo Creek disaster survivors, 55
  in children, 62
  in denial phase, 46
  and diminished interest in activities, 22
  family therapy in, 199
  and feelings of detachment and
    estrangement, 23–24
  information-processing model on, 70,
    71
  in oscillation phase, 46
  psychodynamic therapy in, 152, 154,
    155
  psychoformative theory on, 87, 88
  and psychogenic amnesia, 24
  restricted range of affect in, 22–23

Object relations theory on PTSD, 89–91
  hypnotherapy in, 172
Obsessional style of information
  processing in PTSD, 71–72, 186
  psychodynamic therapy in, 152, 157–
    158
Omnipotence, pathological, in object
  relations theory on PTSD, 90
Oscillation phase of PTSD, 46, 49
  information processing model on, 70,
    71
  psychodynamic therapy in, 152
Outcry phase of PTSD, 46

Panic disorders
  differential diagnosis of, 116
  drug therapy in, 215
Paranoia in PTSD, 31
Parental responses in PTSD of children,
  64–65
Passive role in traumatic event, assessment
  of, 124
Patterning of cues, in behavioral theory
  on PTSD, 76

Personality in PTSD, 41
  antisocial, 118–120
  in maladaptive changes, 49
  splits in
    and hypnotherapy as integrative
      technique, 172, 176
    object relations theory on, 89–90, 91
Phases of PTSD, 46, 152
  information processing model on, 71
  stage theory on, 46–47
Phenelzine therapy in PTSD, 215
Picture drawing in therapy of PTSD in
    children, 206, 209
Plaintiff, forensic evaluation of PTSD for
  agenda of, 130
  ethical issues in, 128–129
  interpretations and conclusions in, 132–
    133
Play therapy in PTSD of children, 205,
    210
Political issues in PTSD, 7–8, 9, 218
Prevention of PTSD, 218–219
Primary symptoms of PTSD, 11–34
Professionals, mental health. See Mental
    health professionals
Propranolol therapy in PTSD, 214, 215
Protective self, in object relations theory
    on PTSD, 91, 176
Psychic numbing in PTSD, 21–25, 26, 55,
    62. See also Numbing of
    responsiveness in PTSD
Psychoanalytic theories on PTSD, 82–84,
    151–152
  in therapy, 151–158
  in groups, 184, 187–189
Psychobiological models on PTSD, 91–94
  arousal symptoms in, 31, 93, 214
  drug therapy in, 94, 214
Psychodynamic theories on PTSD, 82–84,
    151–152
  in cybernetic model, 94, 95
  in information processing model, 72
  in therapy, 7, 145, 151–158
    assessment of patient in, 152–154
    effectiveness of, 158
    goals, phases and priorities in, 155–
      156
    in groups, 184, 187–189
    in hysterical style of information
      processing, 152, 156–157
    in obsessional style of information
      processing, 152, 157–158

Psychodynamic theories on PTSD (cont.)
  in therapy (cont.)
    strategies in, 154–155
Psychoformative theories on PTSD, 87–88
Psychogenic amnesia in PTSD, 24
  hypnotherapy in, 173–174
Psychometric and psychodiagnostic
    testing in PTSD, 111–115
Psychoneurosis in disaster survivors, 56
Psychopharmacological treatment of
    PTSD, 213–216. See also Drug
    therapy in PTSD
Psychophysiological model on PTSD, 91–
    94
  assessment procedures in, 114
Psychosocial theories on PTSD, 72–75,
    84–86
  assessment procedures in, 124, 125–126
  combined with psychoformative theory,
    87–88
  in ecosystemic model, 96
Psychosomatic symptoms of PTSD, 39–40
  in children, 14
  in rape victims, 40, 52
Psychotherapy, dynamic, in PTSD, 7, 145,
    151–158

Radiation exposure of Hiroshima
    survivors, and PTSD, 58–59
Rage in PTSD, 28–30
Rape victims, PTSD in, 8–9
  adaptive resolution of, 53
  behavioral theory on, 76
  cognitive appraisal model on, 53, 54, 80
  course of, 51–55
    disorganization (acute) phase in, 52–
      53, 54
    reorganization (long-term) phase in,
      53–54
    variables affecting, 54–55
  ecosystemic model on, 96
  emotional reactions in, 53
  hypnotherapy in, 175, 176
  impact reactions in, 52
  intercurrent stressors in, 137
  in physical injuries, 54
  problems in assessment of, 135
  psychosocial model on, 74
  self-blame in, 33, 53
  somatic symptoms in, 40, 52
  stress inoculation training in, 7, 166–
    168, 169

Railway spine, 3
Reaction Index, 115
Reality, constructs of, in PTSD, 6
  cognitive appraisal model on, 78–79,
    81, 101
Recollections in PTSD. *See* Memory in
  PTSD
Recovery environment in PTSD,
  assessment of, 125–126
Reenactment of trauma in PTSD therapy,
  6
  in children, 206–207
  in hypnotherapy, 174, 175
Reexperiencing of trauma in PTSD, 16–
  21, 98
  adaptive value of, 20–21
  dreams and nightmares in, 17–18
  in exposure to symbolic representation
    of event, 15, 20–21
  illusions, hallucinations, and flashbacks
    in, 18–20
  recollections in, 16–17
Refugees, Cambodian, PTSD in. *See*
  Cambodian refugees, PTSD in
Regression, in psychoanalytic theories of
  PTSD, 83, 84
Rehearsal techniques in PTSD therapy
  behavioral, 7, 145, 164–165, 186
  cognitive, 187
Reinforcement, in behavioral theory of
  PTSD, 77
Relaxation techniques in PTSD, 186
  in behavioral therapy, 160, 161, 163,
    165, 186
  in hypnotherapy, 173
Reorganization phase of rape-trauma
  syndrome, 53, 54
Representations of traumatic event,
  symbolic, exposure to, 15
  arousal and startle response in, 30
  distress in, 15, 20–21, 30
Repression, learned, in combat-related
  PTSD, 25
Resolution phase of PTSD, 46, 47–49
  adaptive, 47–48, 49
  ecosystemic model on, 103
  maladaptive, 48–49, 50
Resources of patient in PTSD, assessment
  of, 127
Responsiveness to external world,
  numbing of, in PTSD. *See* Numbing
  of responsiveness in PTSD

Revenge fantasies in PTSD of children,
  207, 209, 211, 212
Role confusion in PTSD
  object relations theory on, 90
  psychological theory on, 85
Role in traumatic event, active or passive,
  assessment of, 124
Rorschach tests in PTSD, 111, 112

Schizophrenia, differential diagnosis of,
  120
Screening for PTSD, 108
  questions in, 109
Secondary symptoms of PTSD, 11, 35–42
Seduction theory, 8
Self-blame in PTSD
  in rape victims, 33, 53
  and survivor guilt, 33
    behavioral type of, as adaptive
      response, 33
    characterological type of, as
      maladaptive response, 33
Self-disclosure in PTSD
  and assessment of silent or reluctant
    patients, 122, 136
  in family therapy, 195, 200
  in group therapy, 185
Self-image in PTSD
  in children, 63, 208, 212
  cognitive appraisal model on, 80–81
  and hypnotherapy as integrative
    technique, 176–178
  object relations theory on, 89–90, 91,
    176
  psychosocial-developmental theory on,
    85, 86, 88
Separation anxiety of children in PTSD,
  63
Sexual abuse and assault, PTSD in, 9, 61
  in rape victims. *See* Rape victims, PTSD
    in
Shell shock, 3, 4
Sleep disturbances in PTSD, 27
  in children, 63
  dreams and nightmares in, 17–18, 27.
    See also Dreams and nightmares in
    PTSD
  drug therapy in, 191, 215
  psychophysiologic model on, 93
Social agency response to PTSD,
  assessment of, 125–126

Social influences in PTSD, 23, 24
  assessment of, 124, 125–126
    in forensic evaluation, 130, 132
  cybernetic model on, 95
  in disaster survivors, 47, 56–58
  ecosystemic model on, 96, 97
  and family therapy, 193
  and group therapy, 183
  psychosocial model on, 74, 75, 84–88
Sodium pentathol, in narcosynthesis, 30, 45
Somatic symptoms of PTSD, 39–40
  in children, 14
  in rape victims, 40, 52
Stage theory on reactions to trauma, 46–47
Startle response in PTSD, 30, 45
  behavioral therapy in, 165
Stimulus generalization, in behavioral theory of PTSD, 76
Strengths of patient in PTSD, assessment of, 126–127
  in forensic evaluation, 132
Stress inoculation training in PTSD, 7, 145, 165–169
  in children, 168–169, 205, 211
  conceptualization phase of, 166
  effectiveness of, 169
  as preventive intervention, 219
  skill acquisition phase of, 166, 168
Stressor, traumatic, in PTSD, 5
  assessment of, 124
    in forensic evaluation, 130, 131–132
    and intercurrent stressors, 137
  diagnostic criteria on, 15–16, 116–118
  ecosystemic model on, 96, 97
  psychosocial model on, 72, 73, 75
Substance abuse in PTSD, 38–39
  assessment of, in forensic evaluation, 130, 132
  and problems in psychopharmacological therapy, 215
Subtypes of PTSD, 43–45
Suicidal behavior in PTSD, 32, 36, 37
Survivor guilt in PTSD, 14, 31–33, 59
Symbolic representations of traumatic event, exposure to, 15
  arousal and startle response in, 30
  distress in, 15, 20–21

Symptoms of PTSD, 11–42. *See also specific symptoms*
  anxiety, 37
  arousal, 26–31
  avoidance behavior, 25–26
  in children, 14, 62–63
  death imprint and death anxiety, 37–38
  depression, 36–37
  in DSM-III and DSM-III-R, comparison of, 12–15
  ego functioning changes, 41
  guilt feelings, 31–33
  impulsive behavior, 38
  miscellaneous, 41
  and nature of traumatic stressor, 15–16
  numbing of responsiveness, 21–25
  primary, 11–34
  reexperiencing of trauma, 16–21
  secondary, 11, 35–42
  somatic, 39–40
  substance abuse, 38–39
  time sense alterations, 40

Task completion difficulties in PTSD, 28
Temper control in PTSD, 29
Tension, and somatic symptoms of PTSD, 39–40
  in rape victims, 40, 52
Terrorist attacks, PTSD in survivors of, 23–24
  in children, 24, 32
  guilt feelings in, 32
  stress inoculation training in, 168
Testing procedures in assessment of PTSD, 111–115
  exaggerated responses in, 121
Theories on PTSD, 67–103. *See also specific theories*
  behavioral, 75–78, 159–160
    therapy based on, 159–169
  cognitive appraisal, 53, 54, 78–82
  cybernetic, 94–96, 102
  ecosystemic, 96–103
  future changes in, 219–220
  historical aspects of, 4–6
  information processing, 69–72
  object relations, 89–91
  psychodynamic, 82–84, 151–152
    therapy based on, 151–158
  psychoformative, 87–88

Theories on PTSD (*cont.*)
  psychophysiologic/psychobiologic, 91–94
  psychosocial, 72–75, 84–86
Therapeutic relationship
  ego-supportive interventions in, 146
  in group therapy, 183, 191
    transference/countertransference phenomena in, 184, 187, 188, 189
  in hypnotherapy, 172, 173, 174, 178
  patient-based problems affecting, 149
  therapist-based problems affecting, 149
Therapist. *See* Mental health professionals
Therapy of PTSD, 141–216
  assessment of, in forensic evaluation, 132
  attributional changes in, 145, 146, 148
  avoidance reduction in, 145, 146, 147
  behavioral, 7, 145, 159–169
  in children, 205–212
  common strategies in, 144–146
  crisis theory on, 143–144, 219
  early intervention in, 143–144
  ego-supportive interventions in, 144, 145, 146
  family and couples in, 7, 145, 193–203
  future changes in, 9, 220–221
  group approach in, 183–192
  historical aspects of, 6–7
  hypnotherapy in, 145, 171–180
  narcosynthesis in, 180–181
  normalizing the abnormal, 144, 145, 147–148
  patient-based difficulties in, 149
  preventive interventions in, 218–219
  psychodynamic, 145, 151–158
  psychopharmacological, 213–216
  recurring problems in, 148–149
  therapist-based difficulties in, 149
Three Mile Island residents, PTSD in, 28, 59, 65
Time sense alterations in PTSD, 40
  in children, 14, 24, 40, 62
Transference/countertransference phenomena in group therapy for PTSD, 184, 187, 188, 189
Trust, in PTSD
  in group therapy, 183, 184
  in hypnotherapy, 172, 173, 178

Ventilation phase of family therapy for PTSD, 200

Veronen-Kilpatrick modified Fear Survey, 115
Veterans, PTSD in. *See* Combat-related PTSD
Victimization, PTSD in
  and adjustment disorders, 117–118
  assessment of, 115
  cognitive appraisals in, 54–55, 79, 80–81, 101
  in crime. *See* Crime victims, PTSD in
  hypnotherapy in, 177
  psychodynamic therapy in, 151
  and satisfaction with justice system, 55, 80, 101
  and secondary victimization, 126
Victim-self, in object relations theory on PTSD, 90, 176
Vietnam veterans, PTSD in, 5, 143, 149
  and antisocial personality, 118–119
  arousal symptoms in, 26, 27, 28–29, 30
  avoidance behavior in, 13
  behavioral theory on, 76
    in assessment procedures, 114
    in therapy, 7, 162, 163
  cognitive appraisal model on, 81
  corroboration of data on, 135
  course of, 51
  depression in, 36, 37
  detachment and estrangement in, 23, 24
  and distress in exposure to symbolic representation of trauma, 20, 30
  dreams and nightmares in, 17, 27
    group seminars on, 190–191
  drug therapy in, 215
  DSM-III criteria on, 134
  ego functioning in, 41
  exaggeration and falsification of data on, 121, 136
  family therapy in, 193, 194, 196, 197, 198–199, 203
  flashbacks in, 18, 19
  group therapy in, 183, 184, 185, 187–188, 190–191, 192
  guilt feelings in, 32
  hypnotherapy in, 171, 175, 176
  interactional styles in, 135
  intercurrent stressors in, 137
  interview technique in assessment of, 110
  intrusive symptoms in, 17

Vietnam veterans, PTSD in (*cont.*)
  irritability, anger, and rage in, 28–29,
    30
  Minnesota Multiphasic Personality
    Inventory in assessment of, 113, 121
  object relations theory on, 89–90, 91
  partial, 134
  problems in therapy of, patient-based
    and therapist-based, 149
  psychoformative theory on, 88
  psychometric and psychodiagnostic
    tests in, 111–112, 113
  psychophysiologic model on, 92, 94
  psychosocial model on, 74, 75, 84, 86,
    87–88
  restricted range of affect in, 22–23
  and schizophrenia, 120
  sleep difficulties in, 27, 215

Vietnam veterans, PTSD in (*cont.*)
  substance abuse in, 38–39, 215
Vigilance, increased, in PTSD, 30–31. *See
    also* Arousal symptoms of PTSD
Violence
  feelings of, in PTSD, 28–30
  and PTSD in children, 62
Vulnerability, sense of, in PTSD
  cognitive appraisal model on, 79–80,
    102
  and paranoia, 31

Withdrawal response in maladaptive
    resolution of PTSD, 49, 50
Work history, in forensic evaluation of
    PTSD, 130, 131

Xenia tornado, 57